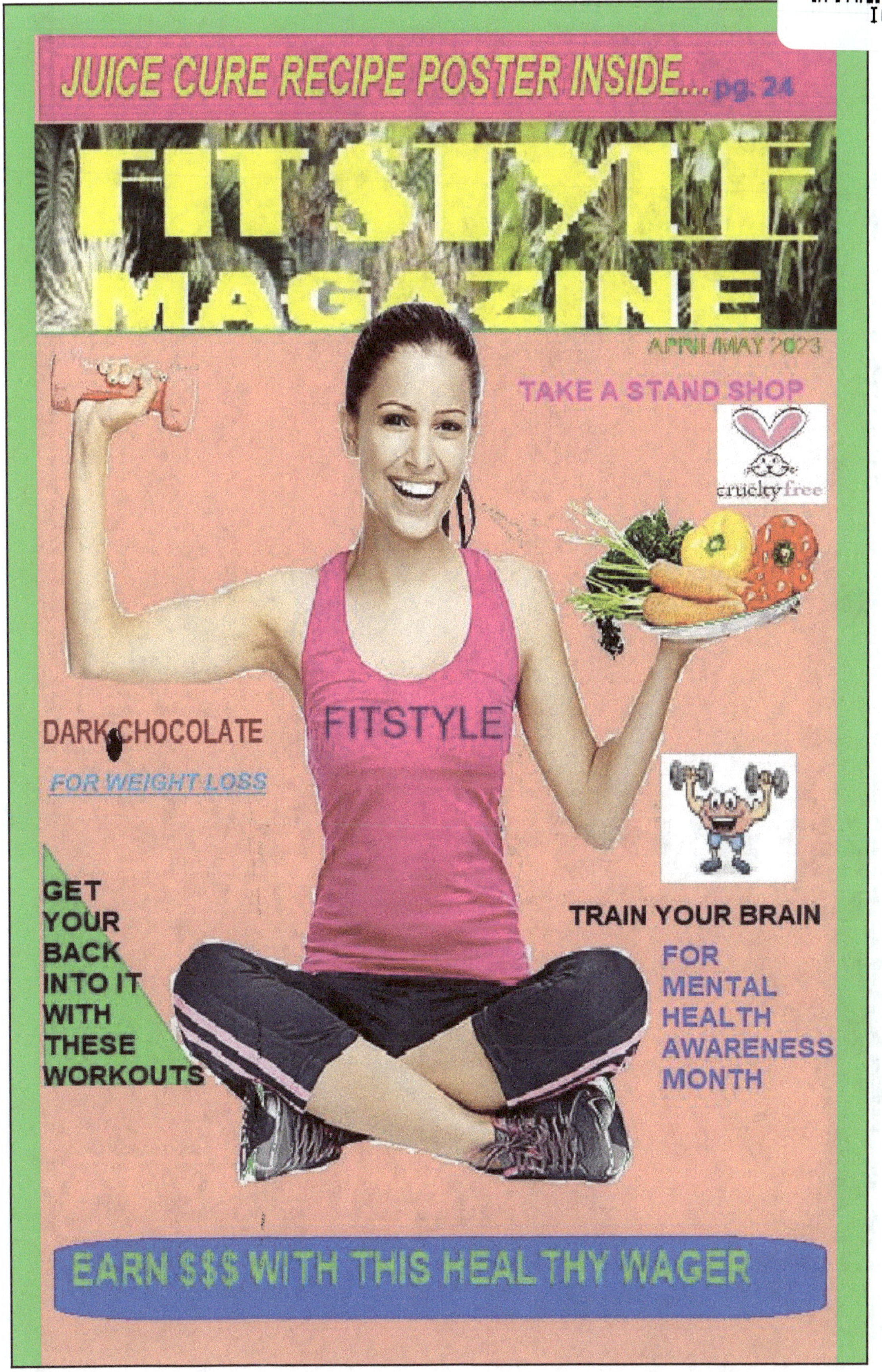

JUICE CURE RECIPE POSTER INSIDE...pg. 24

FITSTYLE
MAGAZINE

APRIL/MAY 2023

TAKE A STAND SHOP

cruelty free

FITSTYLE

DARK CHOCOLATE

FOR WEIGHT LOSS

GET
YOUR
BACK
INTO IT
WITH
THESE
WORKOUTS

TRAIN YOUR BRAIN

FOR
MENTAL
HEALTH
AWARENESS
MONTH

EARN $$$ WITH THIS HEALTHY WAGER

I0838083

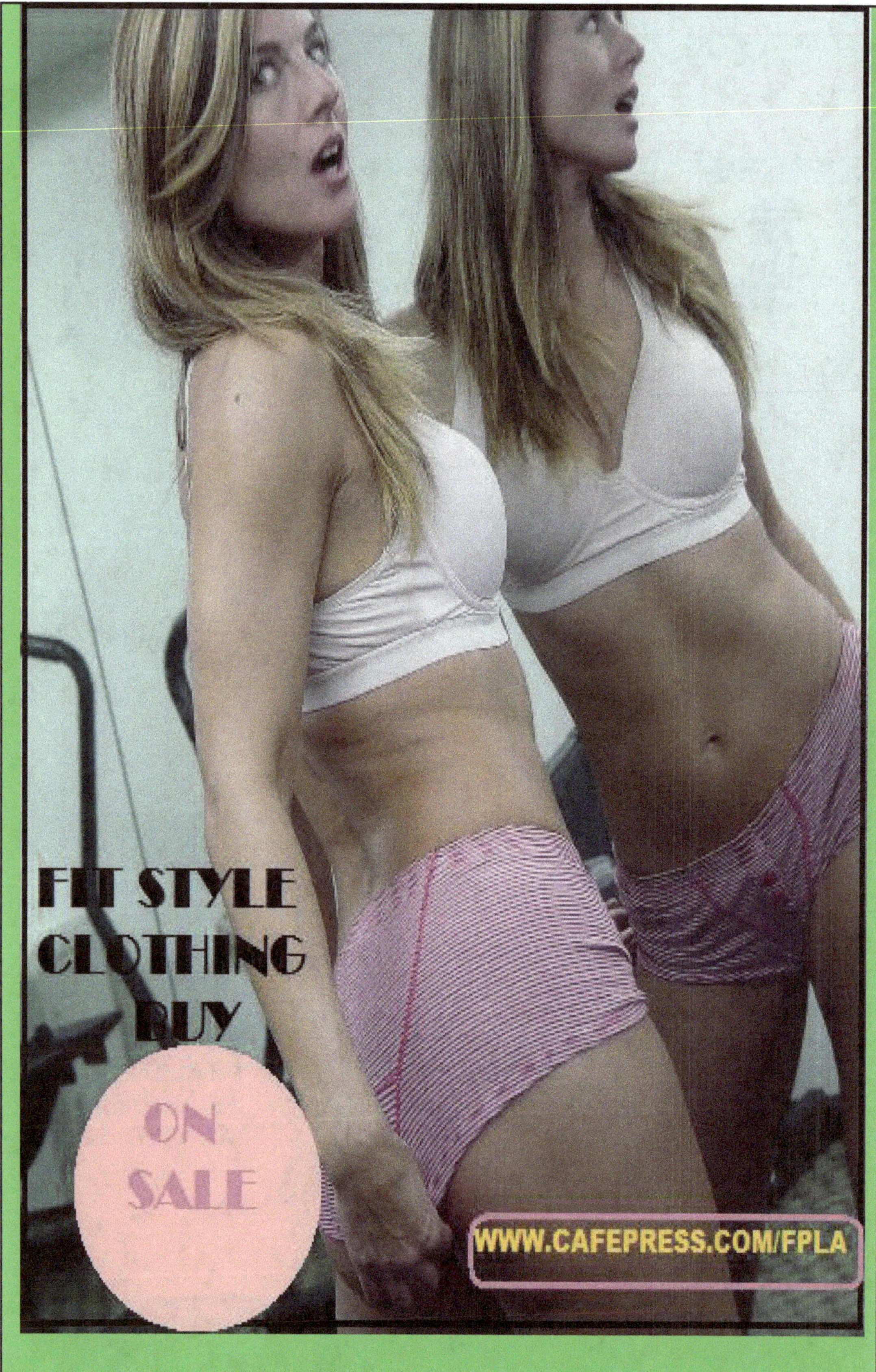
FIT STYLE
CLOTHING
BUY
ON
SALE
WWW.CAFEPRESS.COM/FPLA

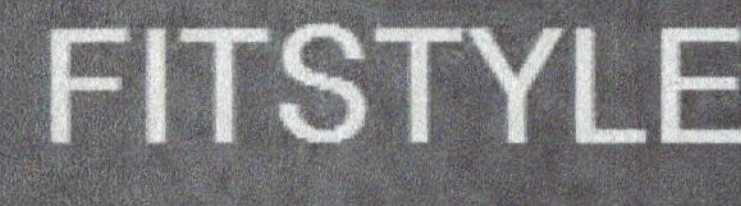
FITSTYLE
BOXERS
WWW.CAFEPRESS.COM/FPLA

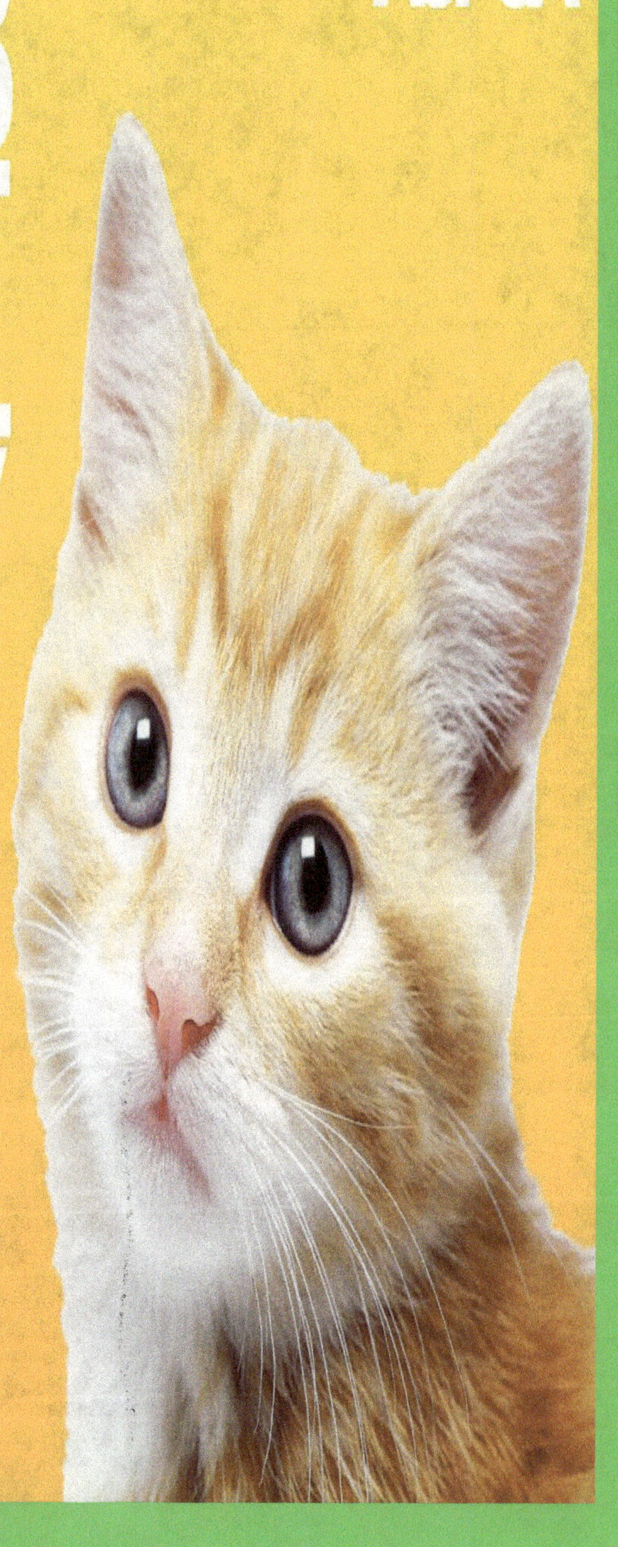
TOP 10 WAYS TO PREVENT ANIMAL CRUELTY
ASPCA
1. Be aware.
2. Learn to recognize animal cruelty.
3. Know who to call to report animal cruelty.
4. Provide as much as information as possible when reporting animal cruelty.
5. Call or write your local law enforcement department.
6. Know your state's animal cruelty laws.
7. Fight for the passage of strong anti-cruelty laws.
8. Set a good example for others.
9. Talk to your kids about how to treat animals with kindness and respect.
10. Support your local shelter or animal rescue organization.

PUBLISHERS

**GFC GROUP
MAGZTER
AMAZON
LULU PRESS**

FOUNDER

Dr. Traci K

CHIEF EDITOR

Dr. Traci K

CONTRIBUTING EDITORS

Ron Anthony

Illustrators/ Photos

PNG EGG
GFC GROUP

CONTACT ADVERTISE

JGFCGROUP@AOL.COM

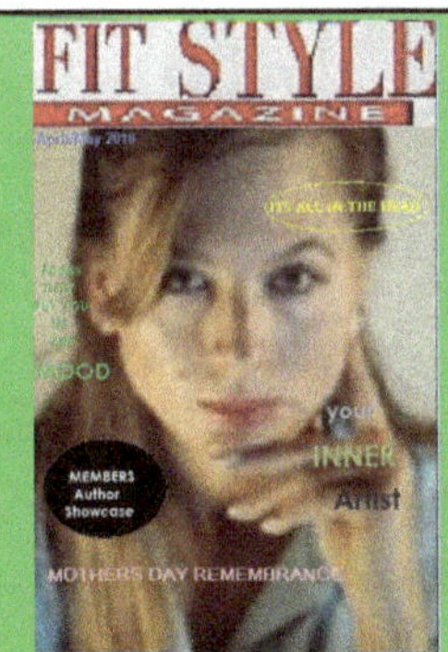
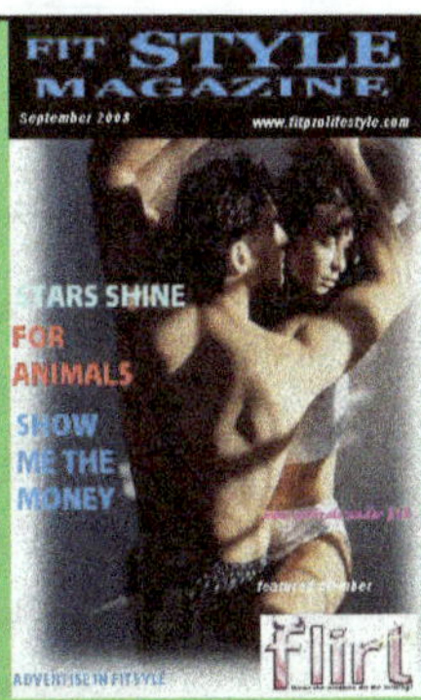
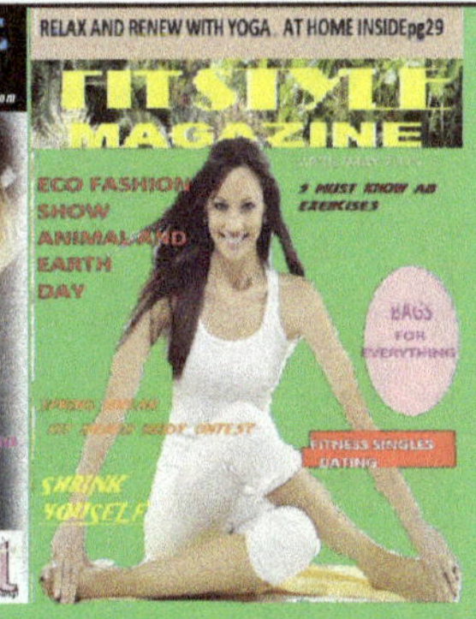

CONTENTS:

10-Pro Diva Network
16-Grow Your Fan Base
18- Fitstyle Your Finance at any age

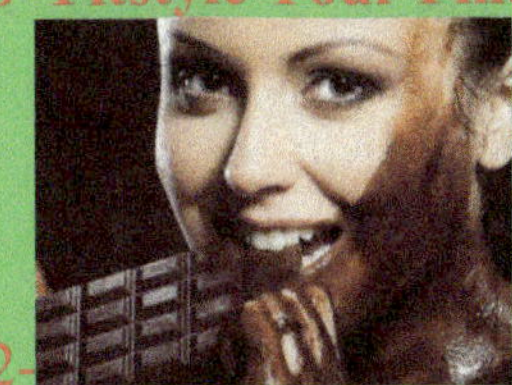

22-
23- Hormone Reset Plan
24- Juice Cure Poster
31- Mothers Day Book Picks   34- Benefits of Oranges
42- Fitstyle Trendy 43- Help Prevent Animal Cruelty
50- $$$ Win Big Real Cash and Prizes with Healthy Wage
74- Earn Extra $ Online
76 Get the Six Pack with these Fitstyle Pros.
 89- Get Your Back Into It with these Workouts

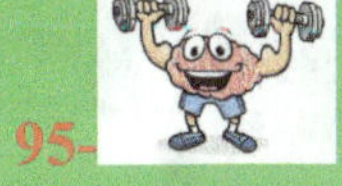

95-   Train Your Brain for Mental Health Awareness Month

SPRING BREAK –FIT BODY CONTEST
Also member news, model highlights, fitstyle trends and
                    fashion
On THE COVER:FITSTYLE TANK TOP FITSTYLE
                    MODEL

advertise or become an ADVERTISER contact
          fitstylemag@aol.com
become a member JOIN www.fitprolifestyle.webs.com
GET THE COLLECTORS EDITTION NOW

Happy Spring Fitstylers,

Well the weather has been quite strange all throughout the globe.   But we are so ready for spring.   I like Spring cause we get to spring forward and watch things bloom.   Birds come to chirp and sing. Squirrels come for nuts and berries. Which is all about this issue.   April is Stop Animal Cruelty. Plus all about wellness and juicing up some healthy recipes.   May brings us Mothers Day in   tribute. Plus Mental Health Awareness Month. So we are going to workout that brain.   If you have any questions or you want to contribute your story email me at fitstylemag@aol.com

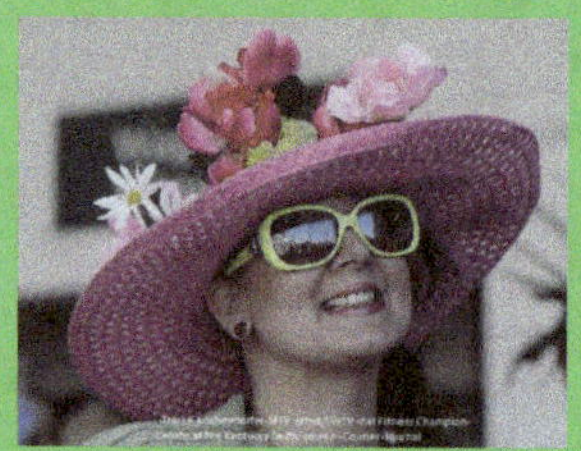

EDITOR : TRACI K

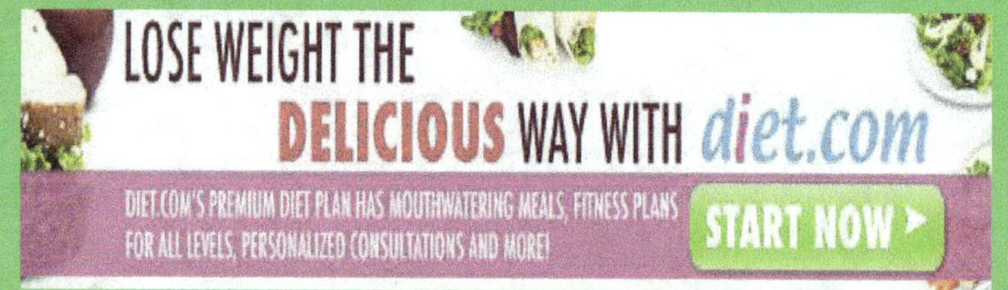

HAPPY EASTER TO YOUR FAMILY AND FRIENDS MAY IT BE A BLESSED ONE

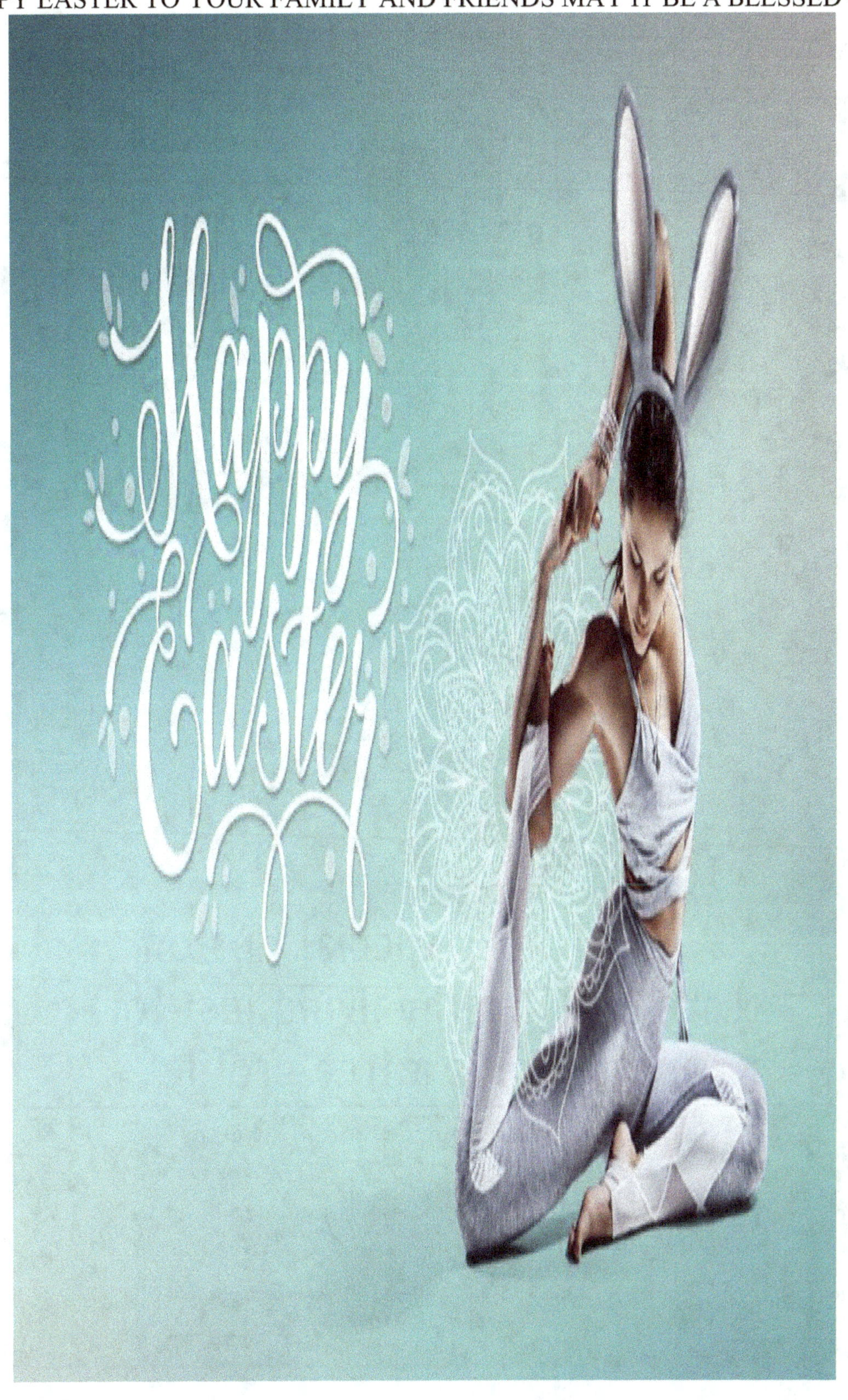

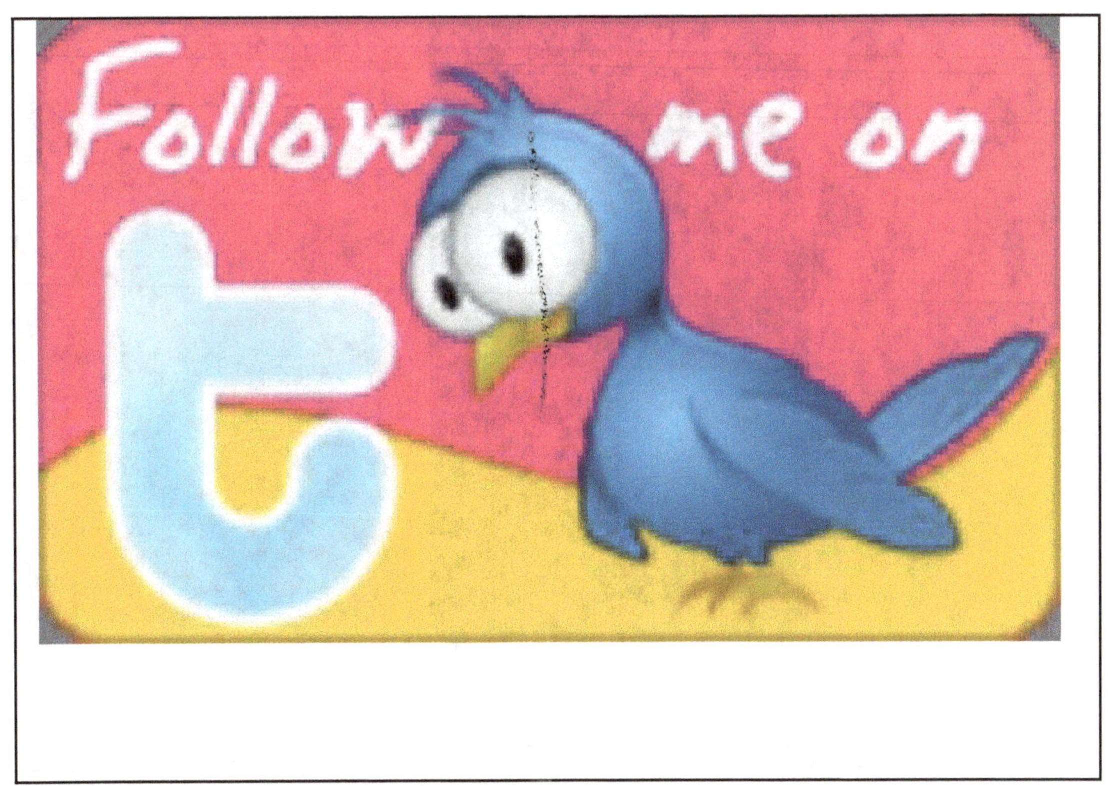

Follow me on

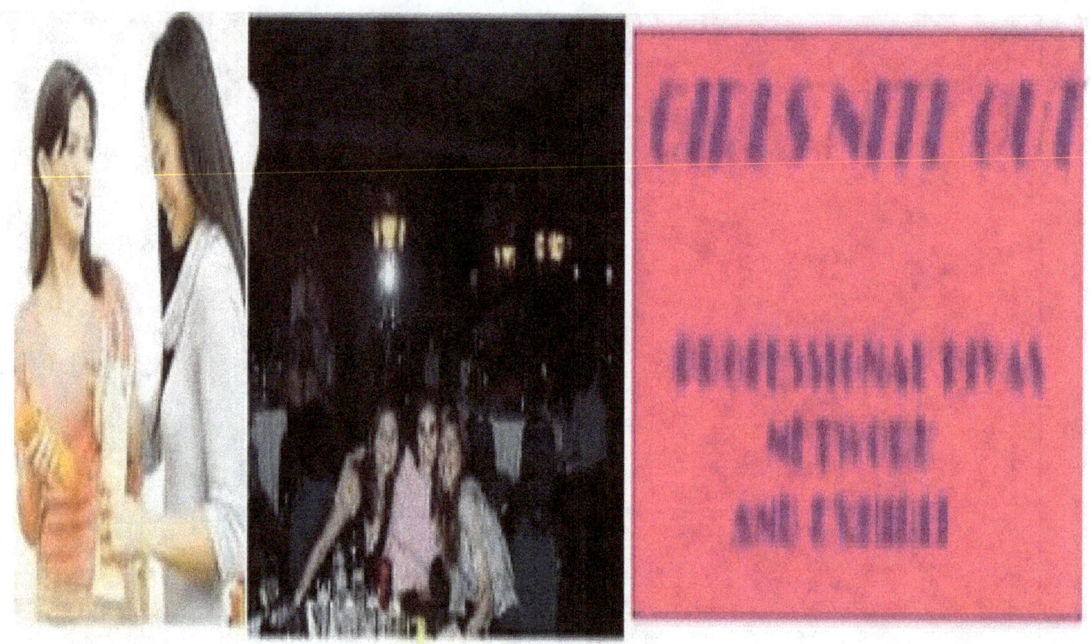

PROFESSIONAL DIVA NETWORK AND EXHIBIT.

Get your diva business or group noticed. Subscribe today for a free trial.
And by showing your support if you purchase one of our Shirts or products we will waive the first month FREE for you and help you advertise your Diva product or be able to come enjoy a night out on us and help be part of a great network.

PROMOTE YOUR GNO GROUP FOR AS LOW AS $25/month

WWW.GROUPS.YAHOO.COM/SUBSCRIBE/GIRLSNITEOUTCAMPAIGNTRIAL

**TO PURCHASE YOUR PRO DIVA STYLE PRODUCT VISIT OUR SHOP
WWW.CAFEPRESS.COM/PRODIVAS**

WWW.FITPROLIFESTYLE.WEBS.COM/BEAUTYWITHOUTCRUELTY.HTM

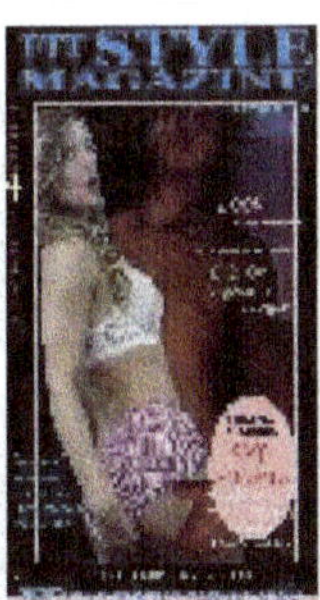

Health Benefits of PINEAPPLES

1: Reduce the blood pressure

2: Support heart health

3: Help to prevent constipation

4: Improve fertility

5: Reduce swelling, bruising, healing and pain associated with injury

6: Help to fight skin damage caused by the sun and pollution

7: Prevent cancer

8: Reduced risk of diabetes

and more

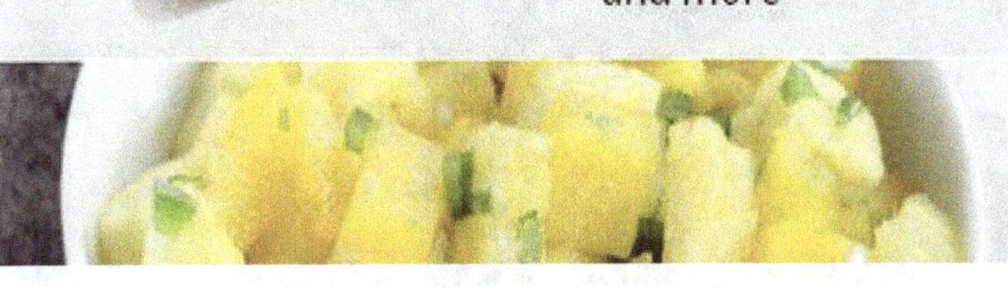

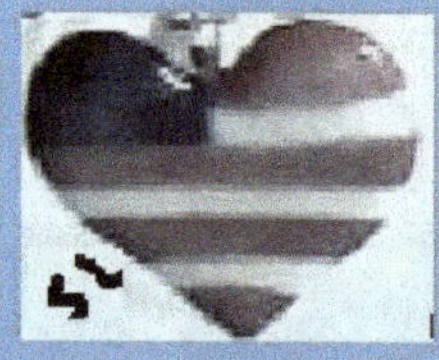

FREEDOM BY LIPINSKI

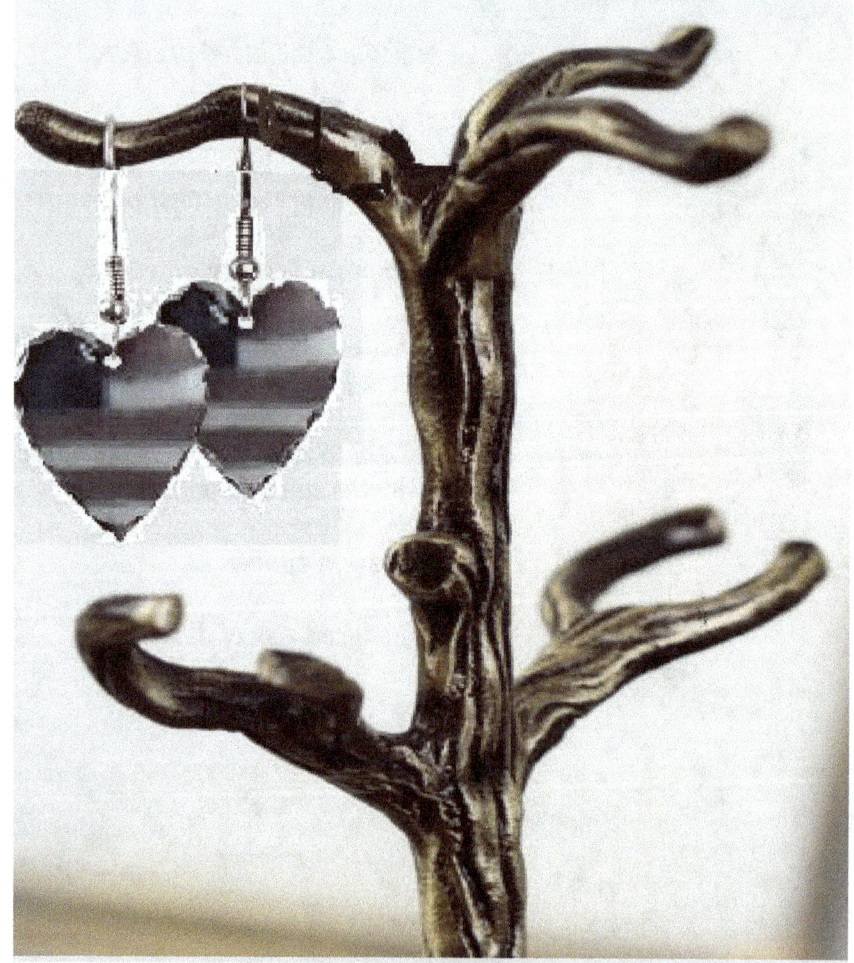

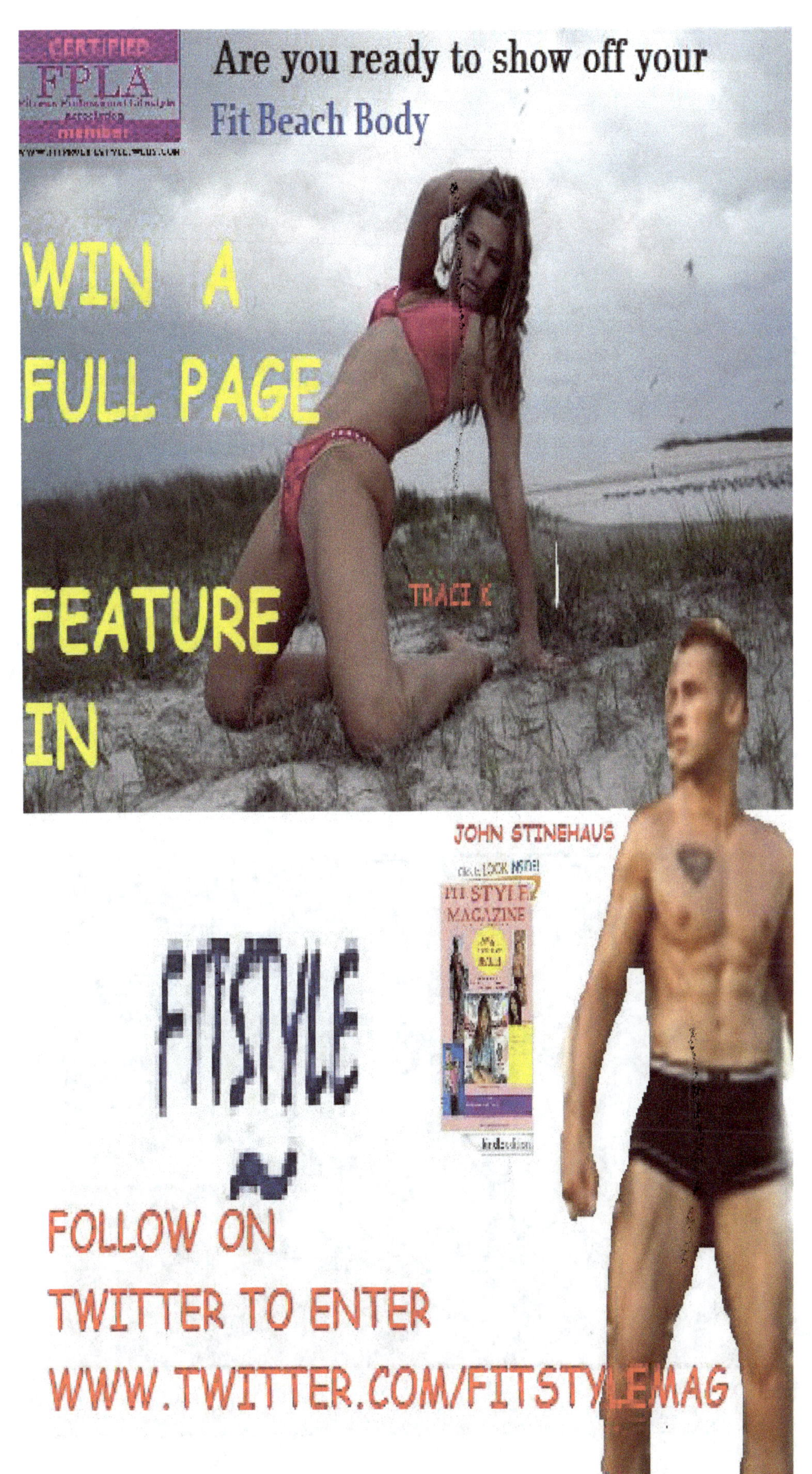
CERTIFIED
FPLA
member
Are you ready to show off your
Fit Beach Body
WIN A
FULL PAGE
FEATURE
IN
TRACI K
JOHN STINEHAUS
FIT STYLE MAGAZINE
FITSTYLE
FOLLOW ON
TWITTER TO ENTER
WWW.TWITTER.COM/FITSTYLEMAG

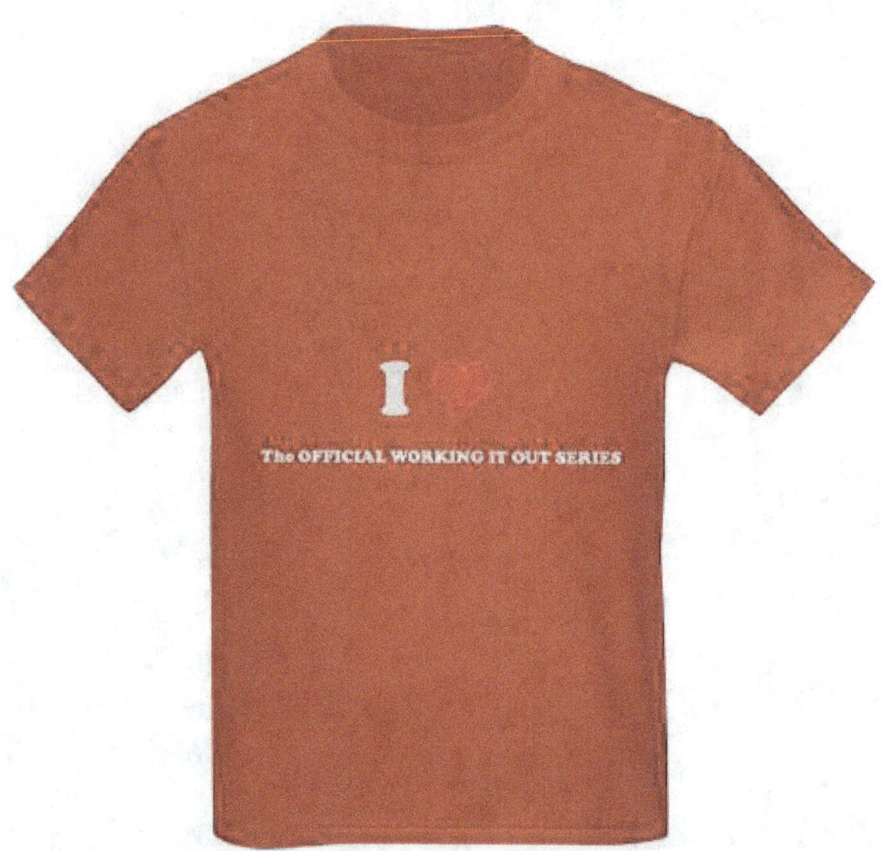
I
The OFFICIAL WORKING IT OUT SERIES

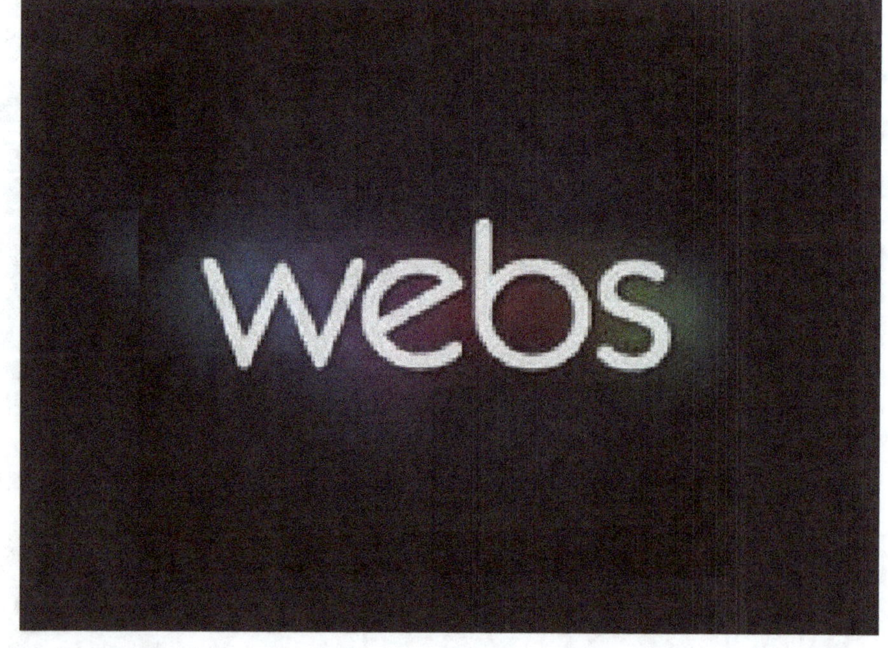
webs

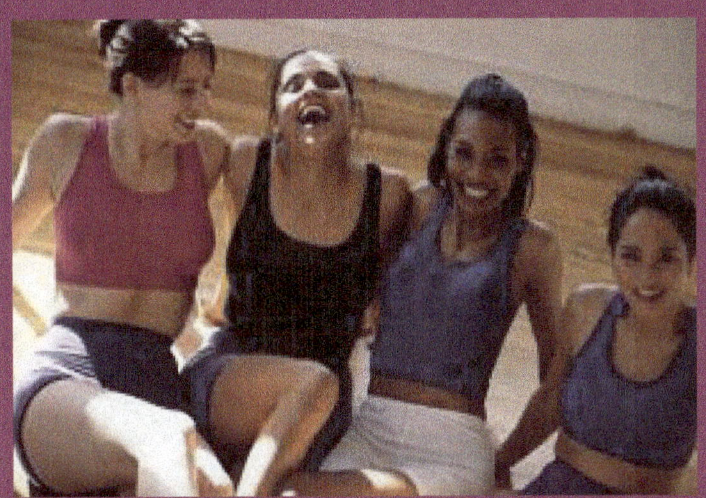

LIFESTYLE AND FITNESS CLASSES
5 DAYS A WEEK
JOIN US TO GET IN ON YOUR CAROLINA PASSES

WWW.FACEBOOK.COM/GROUPS/

Join our group on MEETUP

MEET UP AND GET FREE STUFF
FOR WOMEN ONLY
VIP
TEAM SIGNUP
SPORTS
BEAUTY TIPS
COACHING
MILITARY FUN

learn more when you join the group how to get these

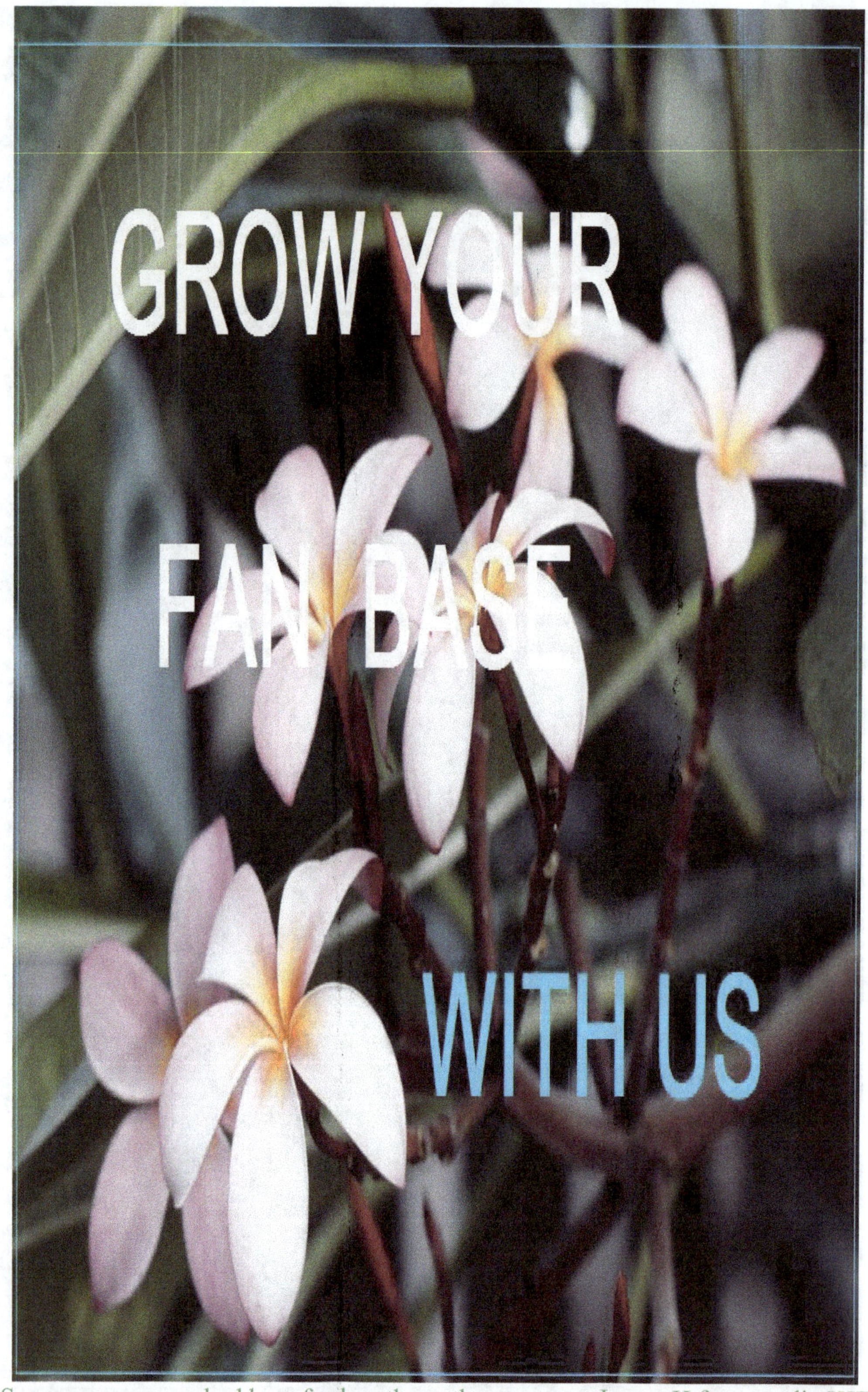

See your sponsored ad here for less than others contact Jen or JJ for a media KIT
jgfcgroup@aol.com

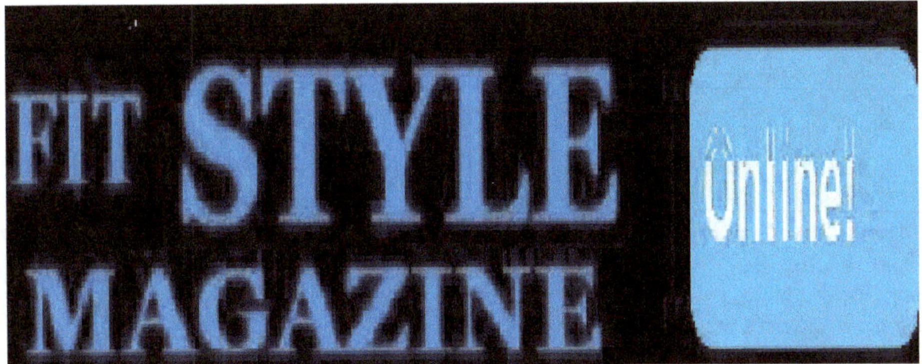

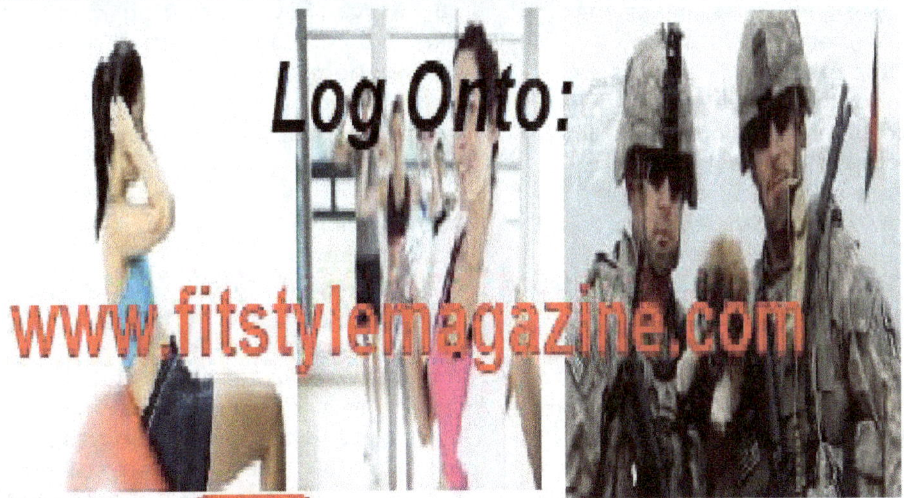

magazine online

Get the magazine online up to weeks before it hits publisher stands

experts online

Real time session with experts and research on health and wellness not in the hard copy

offers online

Get ready for some great deals from sponsors, products, contests, and discounts

featured content

online

You could be featured or check out other stories including model searches

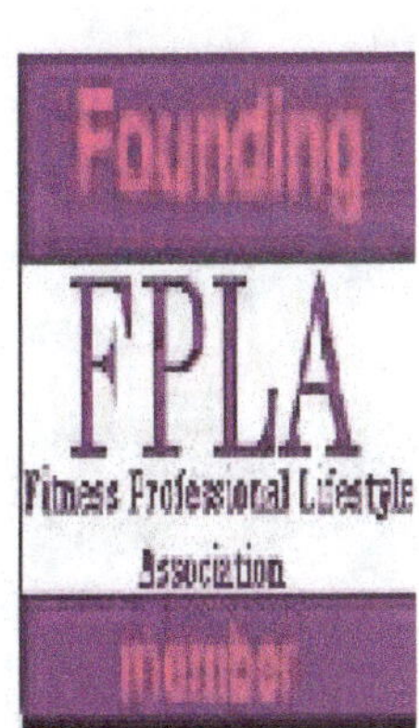

FITSTYLE FINANCE RECAPS

20'S - This is a time of college, fun, life and experiences. But it can also be a time for finding love, marriage and settling down. Don't wait at 18 open up a banking account start putting birthday money, gifts, and savings in it. Establish credit by getting a department card and paying it off every month or fast enought to get your credit established. Some who start jobs make sure you setup a insurance retirement policy with the company and health benefits.

30's- This is when you really need to get your monthly share going and establishing a future for kids, emergency and vacations. If you are working make sure you find what your company offers in IRAs or 401 K that way they can match it after you have worked for them over three years. This will continue on as long as you are employed if you change jobs make sure you find control of it so you don't lose any of the savings in the accounts. Establish a college or emergency fund for your kids or things that happen. Look into investing in real estate cause it is something that grows in value.

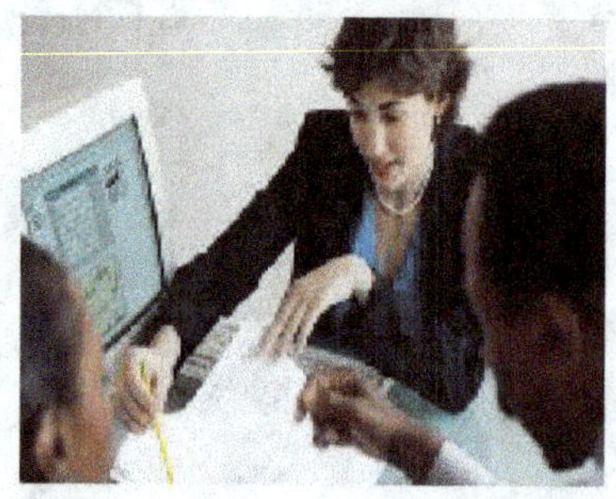

40's - If you have a situation in your life like divorce, medical or other hardship this is where all what you have been doing can come in handy. Your 401 K can be helpful in emergencies or getting back on your feet til you recover. Make sure your IRA is still earning and most of them keep on cause it is a secure savings with good interests this way if you become unemployed, disabled or divorce you can still have something for the future. Check with many resources for help in gathering the best ways to get better credit. creditkarma.com our editors have found does this and helps with disputes and tools. It is all FREE. If you are still raising kids, career and moving fast at this age or dealing with elderly parents. Stocks is something that can be looked at to help grow or be something you want to add. Talk to a financial planner or check sharebuilder.com

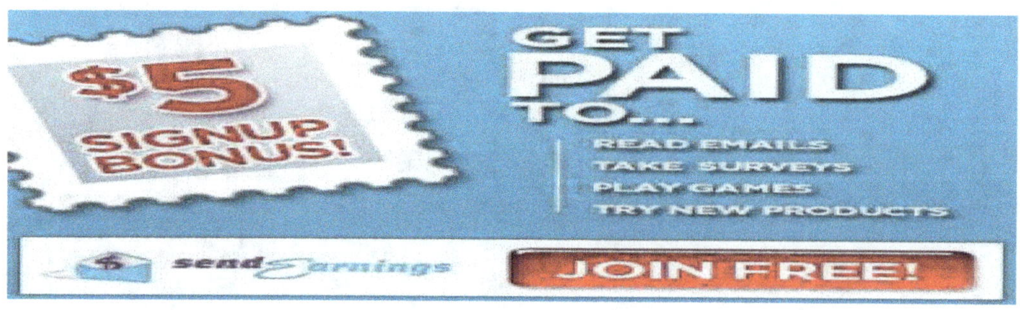

WORKING
IT OUT
APP
APP DOWNLOAD

FITSTYLE SHOOTOUTS – volunteers needed

If you are a model or photographer here is a great way as a member to get your portfolio updated FREE.

Many ways to meet and greet with different shoots and style. From pinups, headshots, body shots, and fun events shots. Want to help us fundraise. And get some great photos to use for you resume...

When it comes to getting out there and being part of a healthy lifestyle community it is about showing others your style in the community...

If you would like to help with volunteering and getting some great free stuff please contact us and help with car washes, photography, clothing...

When you donate these types of things you are helping with getting in shape , developing someone's confidence... and giving them opportunities to meet others and get more out of life

To be part of this....contact us at fitprolifestyle@yahoo.com subject- fitstyle shootouts

TALK TO US
Visit us on face book- logon search fit style
Follow us on TWTTTER   www.twitter.com/fitstylemag
Write the editor a letter at fitstylemag@aol.com
DO YOU HAVE AN ARTICLE YOU WANT TO CONTRIBURE

WE ARE SEEKING ALSO FITSTYLE AMBASSADORS

JUST SIGN UP AT WWW.FITPROLIFESTYLE.WEBS.COM AND BECOME   A MEMBER TODAY

AND SUBSCRIBE.

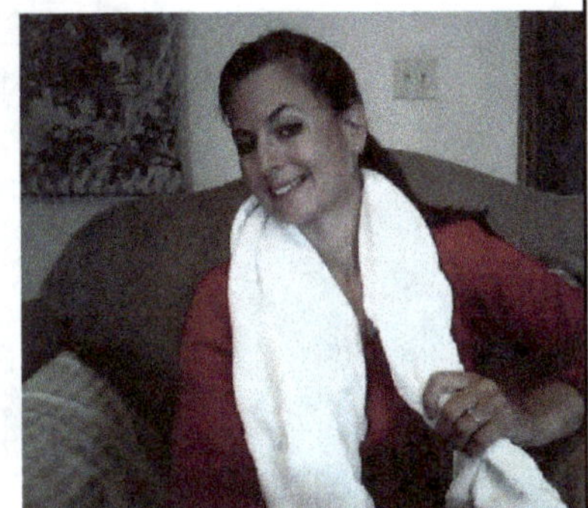

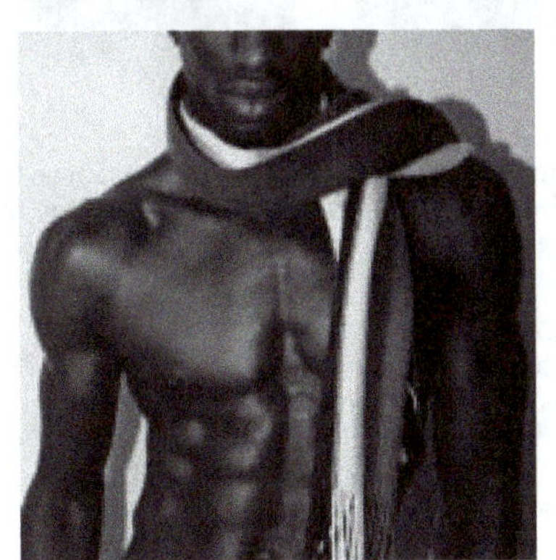

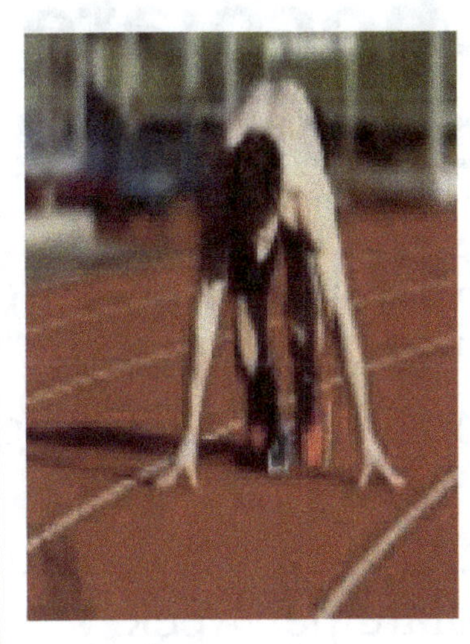

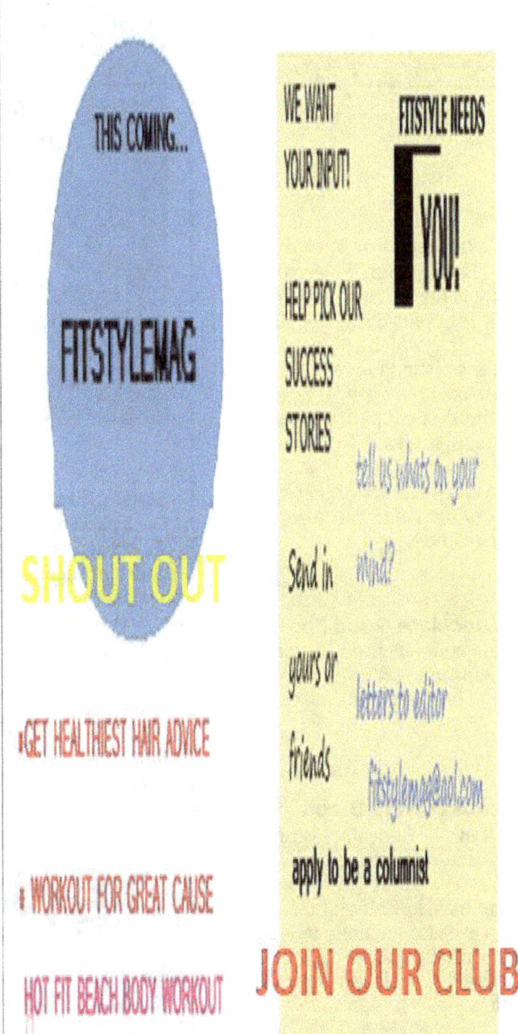

MEMBERS JOIN GET SCENE

FREE SAMPLES, EVENTS AND FUN

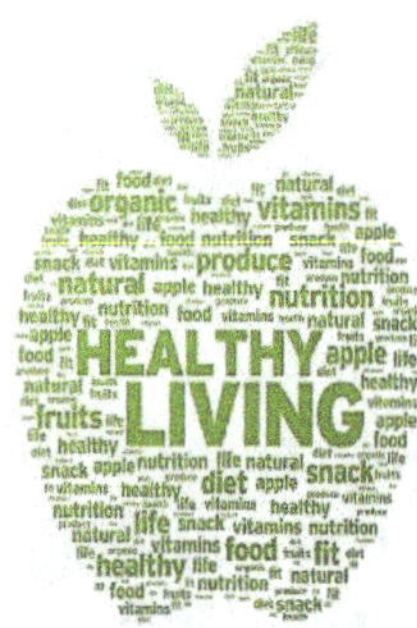

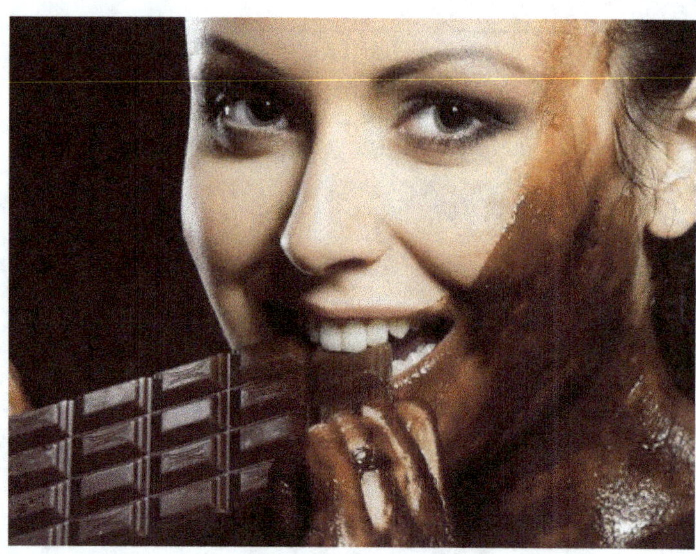

Dark Chocolate For Weight Loss:

Eating a small piece of dark chocolate is the quickest way to kill your cravings plus dark chocolate is high in fiber which will help keep you full & satisfied longer. "Dark chocolate is bittersweet. Whereas sweet stimulates appetite, bitter actually suppresses it."

-Dr. David Katz *MD, MPH, director of the Yale Prevention Research Center*

Dark Chocolate Good For Teeth

Chocolate contains theo-bromine which helps prevent tooth decay by killing the bacteria that causes tooth decay.

Chocolate Lowers Blood Pressure:

Chocolate is full of flavones that improves blood vessel flexibility. The Kuna Indians who are known to have low blood pressure and who are also virtually free of heart disease drink lots of unprocessed chocolate as part of their diets.

Dark Chocolate Makes You Look Younger:

Dark chocolate is high in antioxidants (about 8 times as more than strawberries) which helps protect your skin from sun damage but...This does not mean you can get away with not putting on any sunscreen

Chocolate the Anti-depressant:

Chocolate makes your body release the 'feel good' hormones endorphins & serotonin and believe it or not A study out of the University of Sussex found chocolate to be better than kissing!   "There is no doubt that chocolate beats kissing hands down when it comes to providing a long-lasting body and brain buzz.

Dark Chocolate to Live Longer?

There's no concrete evidence to support this but Jeanne Louise Calment who is the world's longest lived person **Lived to be 122 years old** and she ate 2½ pounds of dark chocolate per week

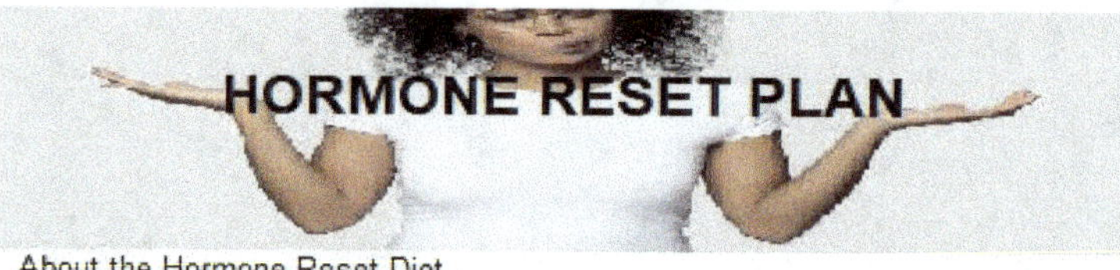

About the Hormone Reset Diet
The guidelines for the Hormone Reset Diet are available in a book by Sara Gottfried titled The Hormone Reset Diet: Heal Your Metabolism and Lose Up to 15 Pounds in 21 Days. It proposes an outline for how to grow new receptors for your metabolic hormones so you feel better and lose weight faster.

The diet claims to help you:

Grow new thyroid receptors to allow you to increase your metabolism
Balance estrogen and progesterone receptors to increase your ability to lose weight
Reset your glucocorticoid receptors so you can better process cortisol and reduce signs of aging
It is also said to boost energy and minimize illness. Some recommendations on the foods to eat and avoid are based on a quiz taken in the book.

The diet is a 21-day program that claims to help you lose 15 pounds within three weeks.

What Can You Eat on the Hormone Reset Diet?

Vegetables: The diet recommends that you eat a pound or more of vegetables a day, choosing ones that are low in starch, high in fiber, and stay below the required 99 grams of carbs. These include:

Bell peppers
Mushrooms
Zucchini
Asparagus
Leafy greens
Organic, Free-Range Eggs and Poultry: According to the diet, non-organic, factory-produced poultry and eggs contain toxins that contribute to hormonal imbalance. For best results, stick to organic and free-range eggs and meats such as chicken, duck, and turkey.

Wild Caught Fish: Wild caught fish is recommended as it does not contain toxins that interfere with hormonal imbalance.

Plant-Based Zero-Calorie Sweeteners: Plant-based zero-calorie sweeteners are Hormone Reset Diet approved as they are low-calorie and more natural than artificial sweeteners. They are also sugar-free and will not increase blood sugar. Examples include:

Erythritol
Stevia
Xylitol

Red Meat: Red meat is eliminated as it contains estrogen that can interfere with weight loss.

Alcohol: Alcohol is thought to cause an increase in estrogen levels.

Sugars: Sugar leads to insulin resistance which causes weight gain. People on the Hormone Reset Diet should avoid consuming any foods with added sugar, as well as fruit and juices.

Artificial Sweeteners: Artificial sweeteners are considered toxic and should be eliminated from the Hormone Reset Diet. They include:

Aspartame
Sucralose
Saccharin
Fruit: Fruit contains fructose, which Gottfried claims interfere with the hormone leptin that helps control appetite. The only fruits permitted on the Hormone Reset Diet are avocado and lemon.

Caffeine: Caffeine increases levels of the stress hormone cortisol.

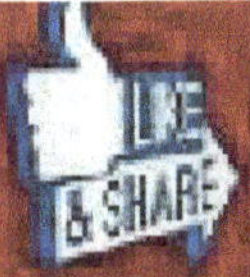

Juice Cure

COLD →
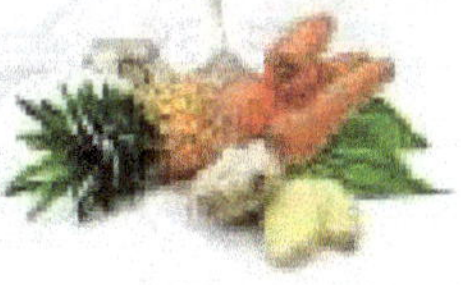
Carrot, Pineapple,
Ginger, Garlic

DEPRESION →
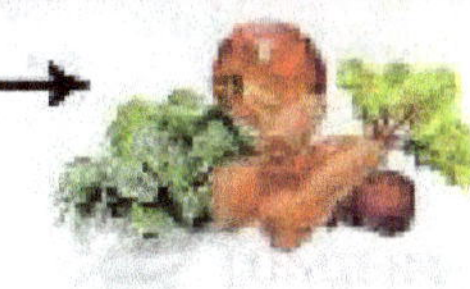
Carrot, Apple,
Spinach, Beet

HEADACHE →
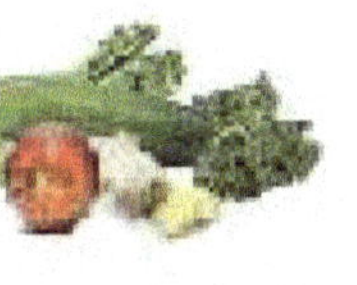
Apple, Cucumber,
kale, Ginger, Celery

DIABETES →
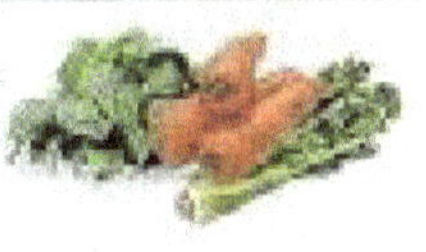
Carrot, Spinach,
Celery

ULCER →
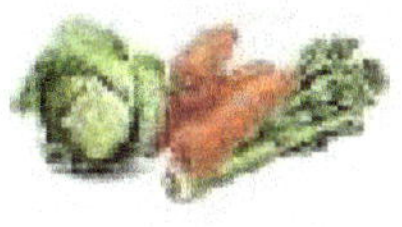
Cabbage, Carrot,
Celery

ASTHMA →
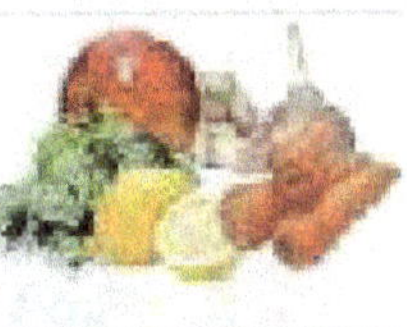
Carrot, Spinach,
Apple, garlic, Lemon

HIGH B.P →
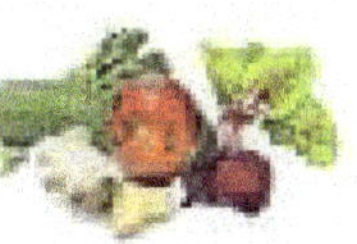
Beet, Apple, Celery,
Cucumber, Ginger

ARTHRITIS →
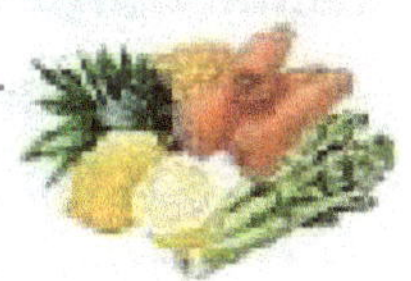
Carrot, Celery,
Pineapple, lemon

KIDNEY DETOX →
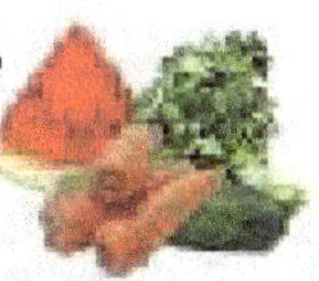
Carrot, Watermelon,
Cucumber, Cilantro

KIDNEY STONE →
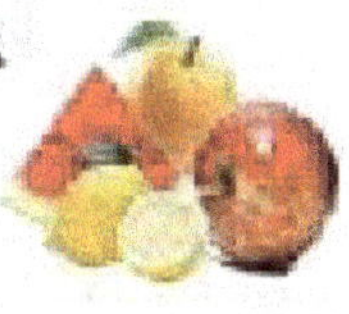
Orange, Apple,
Watermelon, Lemon

EYES →
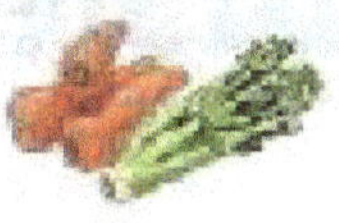
Carrot, Celery

STRESS →
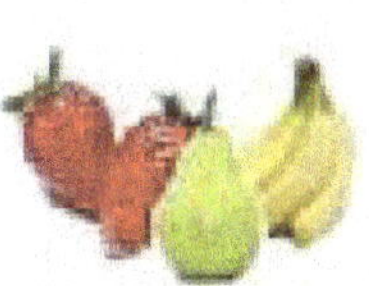
Banana, Strawberry,
Pear

CONSTIPATION →
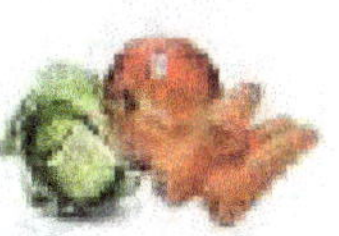
Carrot, Apple,
Fresh Cabbage

FATIGUE →
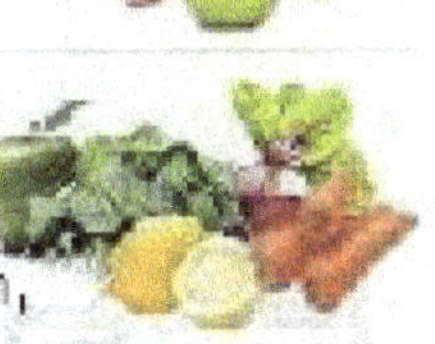
Carrots, Beets,
Green Apple, Lemon,
Spinach

HANGOVER →
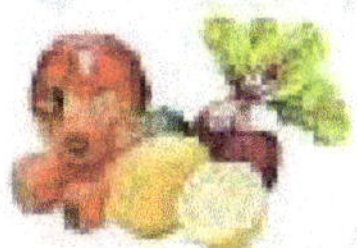
Apple, Carrot,
Beet, Lemon

MEMORY LOSS →
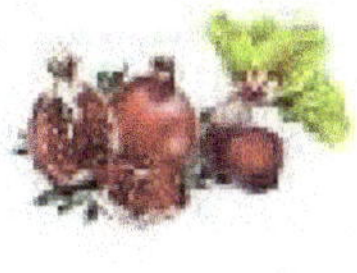
Pomogranate, Beets,
Grapes

NERVOUSNESS →
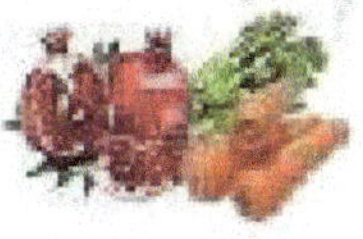
Carrot, Celery,
Pomogranate

INDIGESTION →
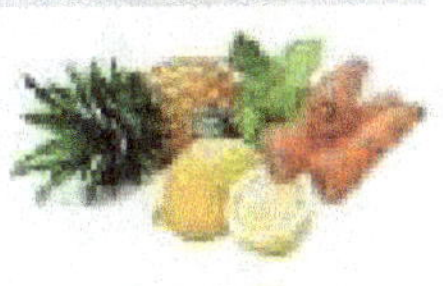
Pineapple, Carrot,
Lemon, Mint

Weight Training for Children?

Most doctors avoid children to start weight training caues it can stunt bone growth. University of Mass. Dr. Avery found in a study that children develop stronger doing more reps 13-15 with light weights instead of low reps. suggestion playground monkey bars or a jungle gym

Weight Training for Weight Loss

We all know someone who has lost a lot of weight in friends or family members. If you notice those who lose weight will have more starved look. If you want to have a healthy firm form. Studies say to lose weight gradually. Like 1-2 a week. Use resistant weights to boost the metabolism at rest and it will have create a more glowfully firm look instead of the starved look

Are Squats SAFE?

Squats when done safely and the right way can help build muscle around the knees and thigns to protect. Plus based on FPLA allow more pep in the step or more spring.

The Belly
We all have ab muscles; it's the fat on top of the stomach that keeps them from showing. Studies have suggested that too much cortisol could be a major factor behind the accumulation of stomach fat. Holy basil is an Indian herb that helps maintain healthy cortisol levels and is commonly taken in capsule form. Foods for reducing cortisol include spinach, citrus, nuts, beans and barley.

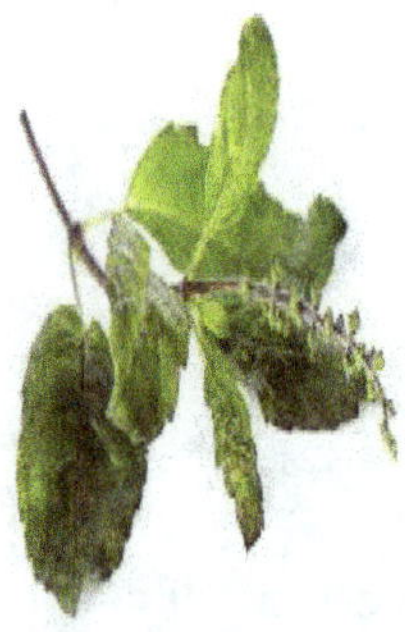

The Back
Fat on the back and upper trunk is less common than stomach fat but equally as challenging to take on. It's also a likely indication that you have high insulin levels. Foods containing conjugated linoleic acid such as milk, yogurt, cheese and beef will help. You should also lean toward whole-grain options and green vegetables.

Hormone-Reset Plan

Try the following hormone-reset recipes

Goat Yogurt and Blueberry Smoothie – Serves 1
Ingredients

    1 serving whey protein isolate
    1/2 cup plain goat yogurt
    1/2 frozen banana
    1/2 cup frozen blueberries
    1 tbsp. chia seeds
    1/2 cup water

Directions
Combine all the ingredients in a blender and purée on high speed until smooth.

Crispy Chicken and Lettuce Wraps – Serves 1

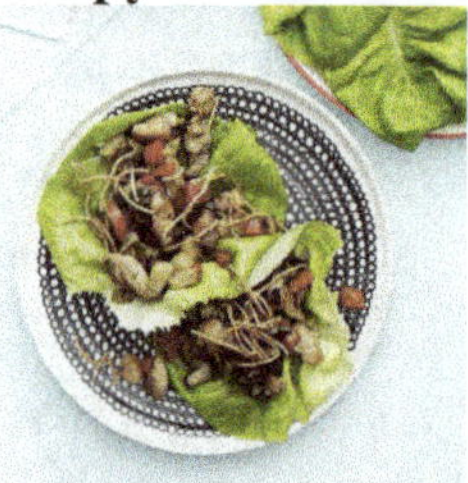

Ingredients

    1 small green apple, diced (unpeeled)
    1/4 cup diced red bell pepper
    1/4 cup diced cucumber
    1 tbsp. finely chopped red onion
    1 boneless skinless chicken breast
(approximately 4 to 5 oz. each), cooked and diced
    1/4 cup low fat Greek yogurt
    2 tsp extra-virgin olive oil
    Salt and pepper to taste
    1 small head of lettuce (4-5 leaves)

Directions
In a bowl combine all ingredients except for the lettuce. Chill for 1 hour. Place the chicken mixture inside each lettuce leaf, roll into cylinders and serve.

If you suffer from belly fat, you can also find how to lose stubborn belly fat for good without counting

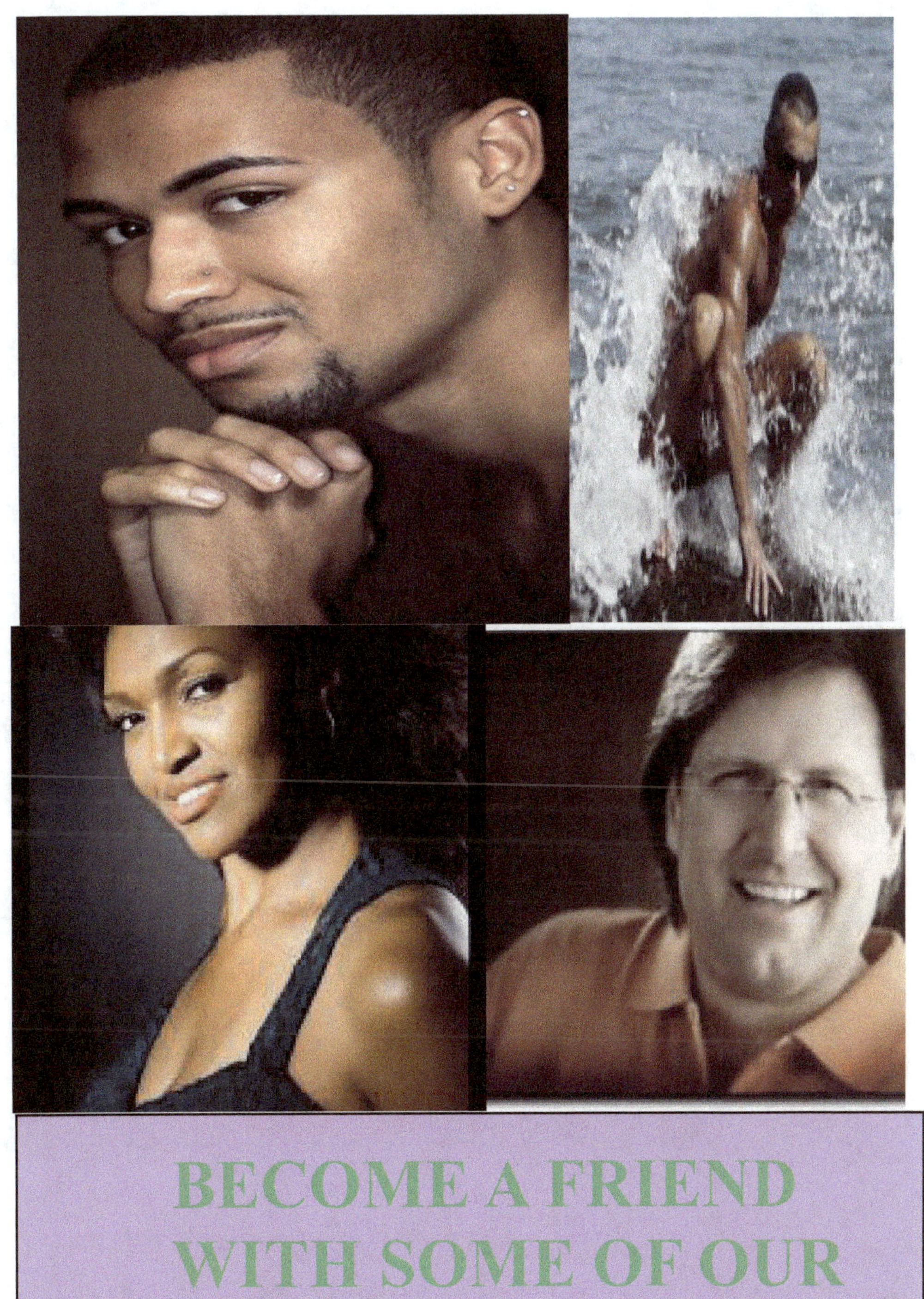
BECOME A FRIEND
WITH SOME OF OUR
MEMBERS

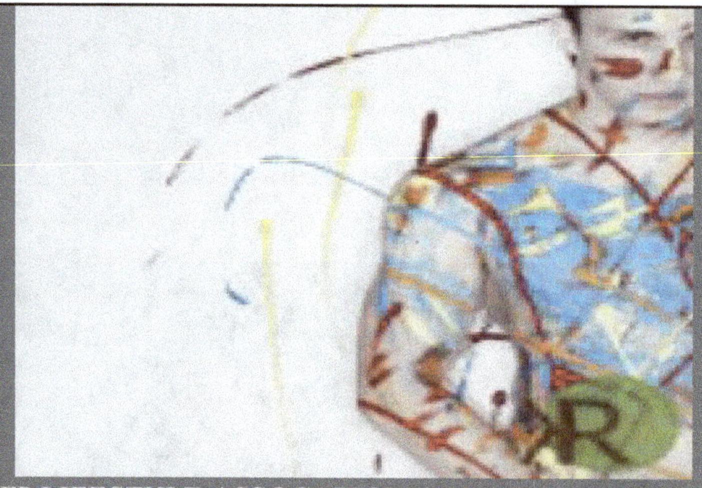

FP LIFESTYLE ASSOCATION AWARDS
CALL FOR NOMINATIONS.
SUBMIT YOUR NOMINATIONS TODAY!
FPLA BOARD is inviting you to join us as a member and nominate and recognize your favorite fit or lifestyle pro...to honor with our benefit online and coming up this year.
IF YOU WOULD LIKE TO NOMINATE OR DONATE SOMETHING IN HONOR OF YOUR FAVORITE PRO…here is your chance and help FPLA.   Raise money The funds will also provide capital items for awards, and also equipment, expenses and club improvements so that we can continue to support our online tools and build … along with enjoying events and fun things to do. And test our skills…
To show your inner artist and help out register your company, team or individual by contacting the director VA at emailing
gofigureliveadvice@yahoo.com

WWW.FITPROLIFESTYLE.WEBS.COM
OR CALL AND GET IN ON THE HOTLINE LEAVE NAME ,
LOCATION AND MESSAGE
HOSTED BY OUR FOUNDER

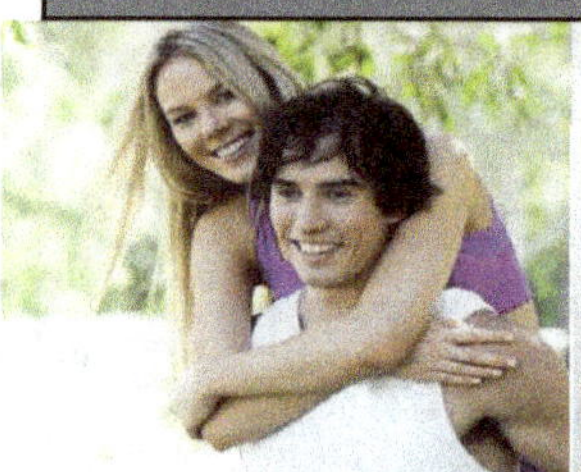

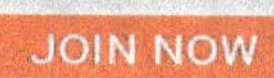

...

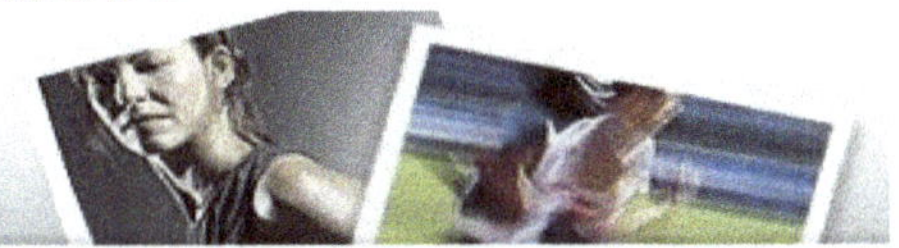

EDITORS PICK…..GOT A BOOK YOU WANT SHOWCASED JOIN GO PRO BE A MEMBER $25 MOTHERS DAYS SECTION THESE AUTHORS HAVE WON AWARDS PLEASE BUY THEM AND SHARE.

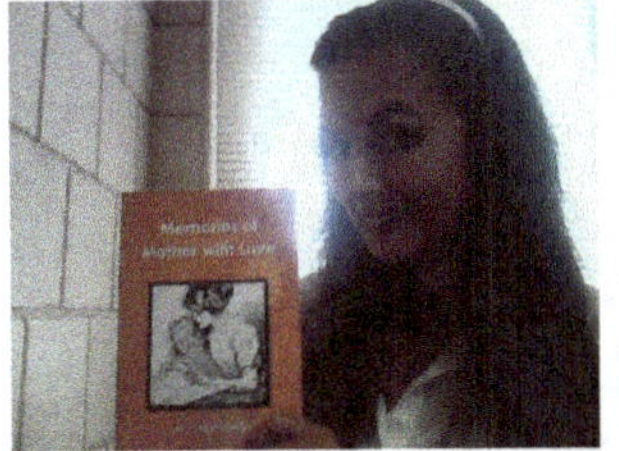

MEMORIES OF MOTHER WITH LOVE BY TRACI K SHOOP

This book is a memorabilia of women in our lives and created by our editor to showcase memories of mothers everywhere.   It is a great gift to give to the special women in your lives. It comes with even added pages to continue those journaled memories.   Please purchase this book today and money from these books goes to families like our editors who have suffered from or died from mental diseases like dementia or PTSD.   You can purchase this book here.

Lulu or Amazon.

FROM MY MAMA'S KITCHEN BY JOHNNY TAN

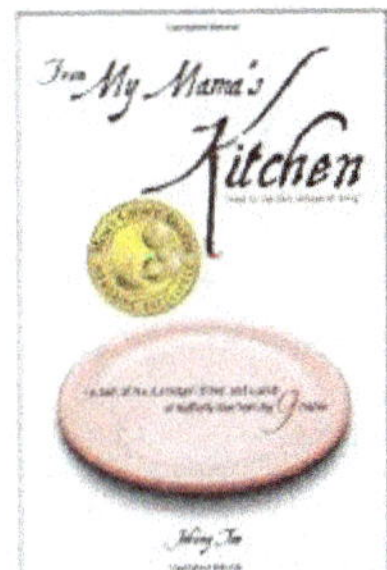
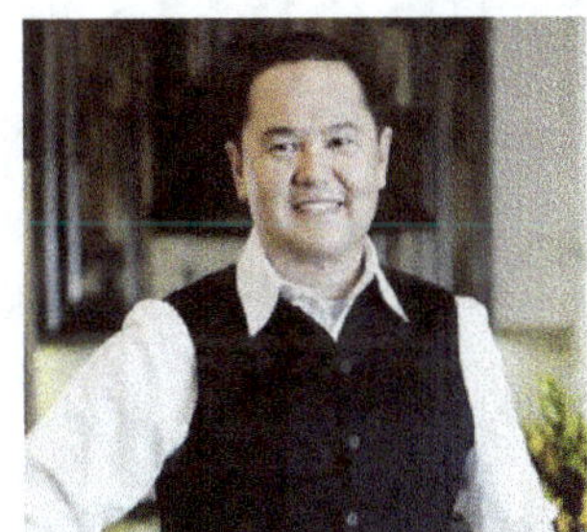

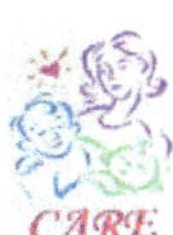

Brought in relation and created by Salvation Army...
Where help with tips for women who are going through hard times and abuse...
Give them resources to get back on their feet again and their family…this program is a great thing.   To learn more about Salvation Army and the Care program visit their website.

FEATURED FPLA MEMBER

RICH PUTNAM
MEMBER ID   108781441 SINCE 2010ADD HIM AS A FRIEND
WWW.FITPROLIFESTYLE.WEBS.COM

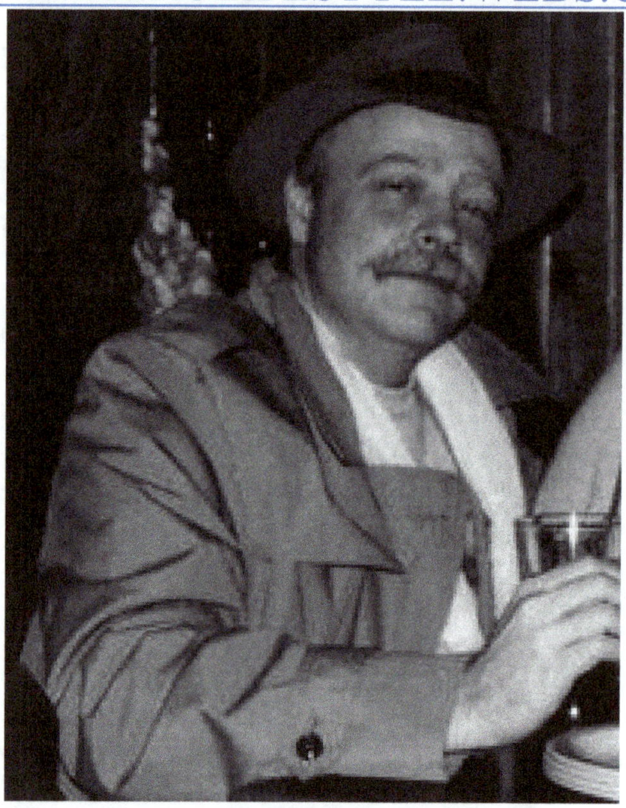

WRITER AND BEEN A LIMITED MEMBER SINCE 2010
FROM DES MOINES , IA

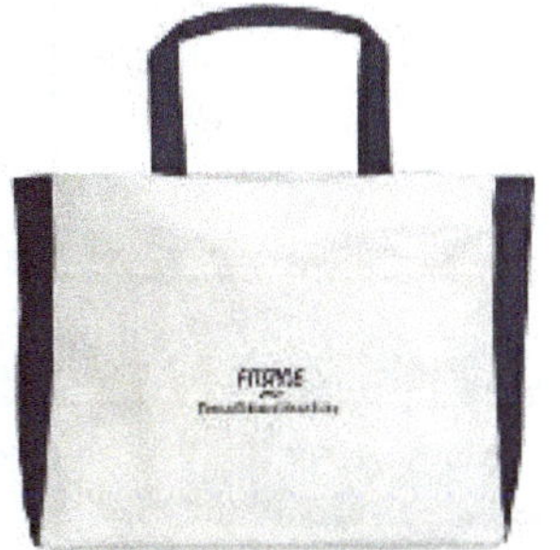

MENS POLO FITSTYLE SHIRT

SHOWING YOUR FIGURE IS FITSTYLE... WITH COZY SNAP UP FITTED TOPS FOR MEN AND FOR YOUR PET TOO.

WHILE STAYING COTTON FRESH WITH A THONG...

WWW.CAFEPRESS.COM/FPLA

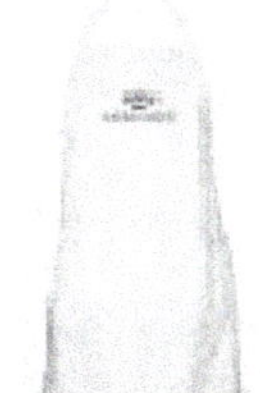

BEACH TOTE

APRON

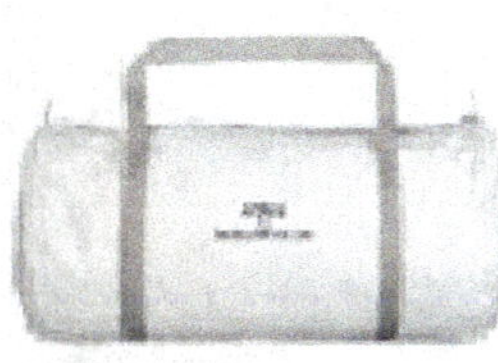

GYM BAG

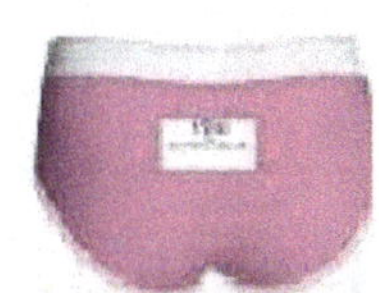

WOMENS BOY BRIEF

THE SEXIEST COTTON WEAR- EVER!

IF YOU LOVE UNDERTHINGS....AND WANT TO STAY FIT AND STYLISH. THESE DESIGNER LINE OF FITSTYLE WILL SURE TO KEEP IT. FROM YOUR POLOP SHIRTS TO THE SEXY WOMENS BOY BRIEF....TO HITTING THE GYM THEN COMING HOME AND COOKING A HEALTHY DINNER.   ALL 100% COTTON AND UNDER $50 TO INCLUDE COLORS TO CHOOSE FROM...

10 Incredible Health Benefits of Oranges

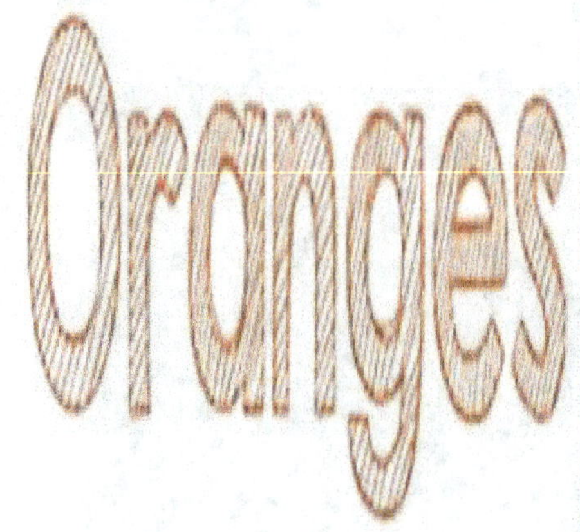

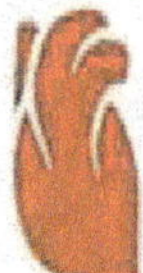

Heart Health
Herperidin's in oranges help lower blood pressure and folate protects against cardiovascular disease

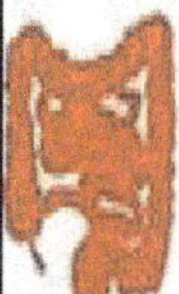

Digestive Health
Vitamin C helps prevent ulcers and fibre ensures a healthy colon

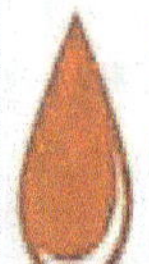

Cholesterol-Lowering
Contain limonin, which helps reduce LDL, or "bad" cholesterol

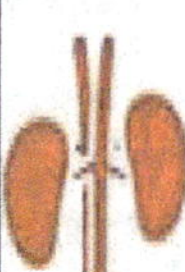

Kidney Support
Help prevent kidney stones & efficient filtering of toxins

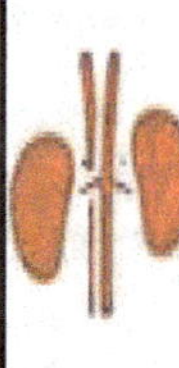

Anti-Cancer
Studies have shown cancer-risk reductions in over 40-50% of individuals who consumed citrus fruits! Contain potent anti-carcinogens to prevent proliferation of cancerous cells.

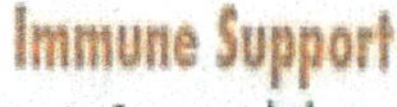

Immune Support
High vitamin C content helps to steer away nasty bugs, bacteria & viruses. Prevents colds, flus & ear infections

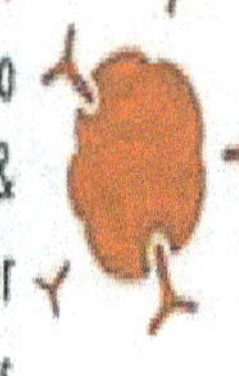

Alkalizing
Rich in alkaline minerals to help balance body pH

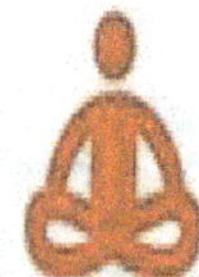

Healthy Skin
Contain essential vitamins & minerals for beautiful, problem-free skin

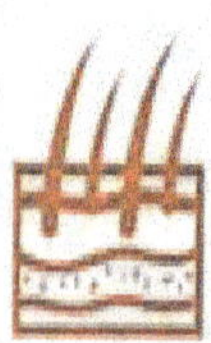

Anti-Inflammatory
Oranges help prevent free-radical damage, which normally triggers the inflammatory cascade

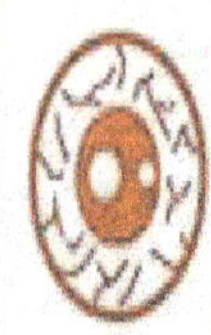

Vision Protection
Loaded with carotenoids, oranges help prevent night blindness & macular degeneration

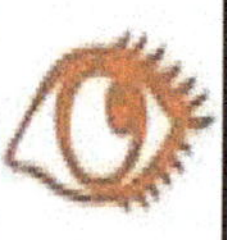

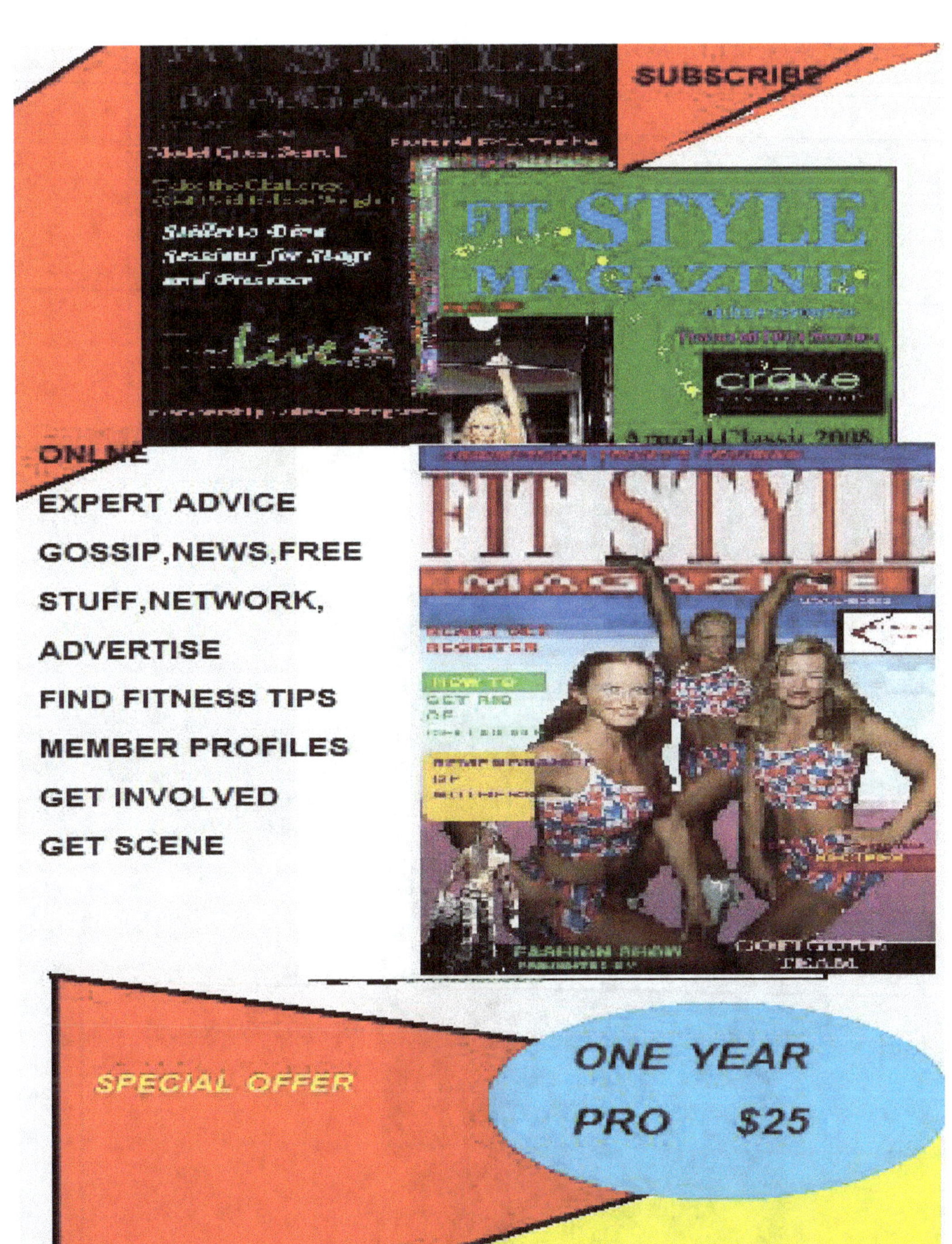

ONLINE

EXPERT ADVICE

GOSSIP,NEWS,FREE

STUFF,NETWORK,

ADVERTISE

FIND FITNESS TIPS

MEMBER PROFILES

GET INVOLVED

GET SCENE

SPECIAL OFFER

ONE YEAR

PRO $25

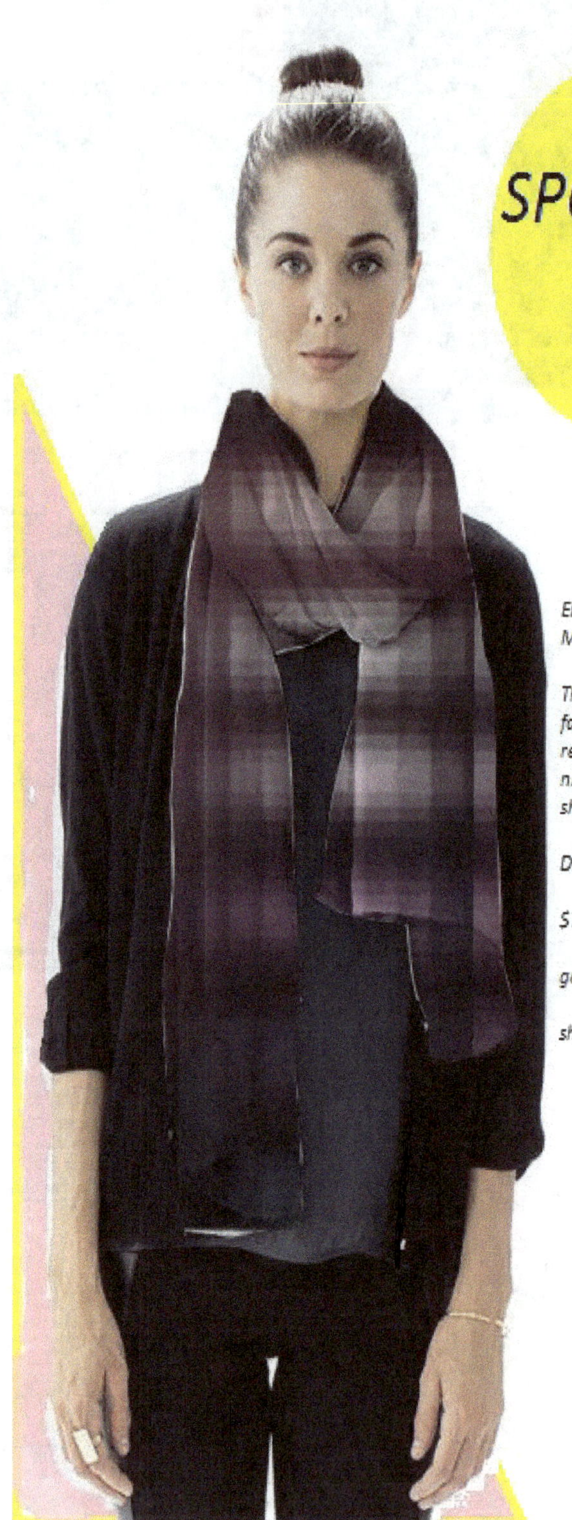

EDM
MODAL SCARF

This scarf made with soft, luxurious fabric features the artist's representation of that effervescent nightlife feeling. Dancing and shimmering all night long.

DESIGNER TRACI K*

$75

get 20% off by going to

shopvida.com/collections/traci-k

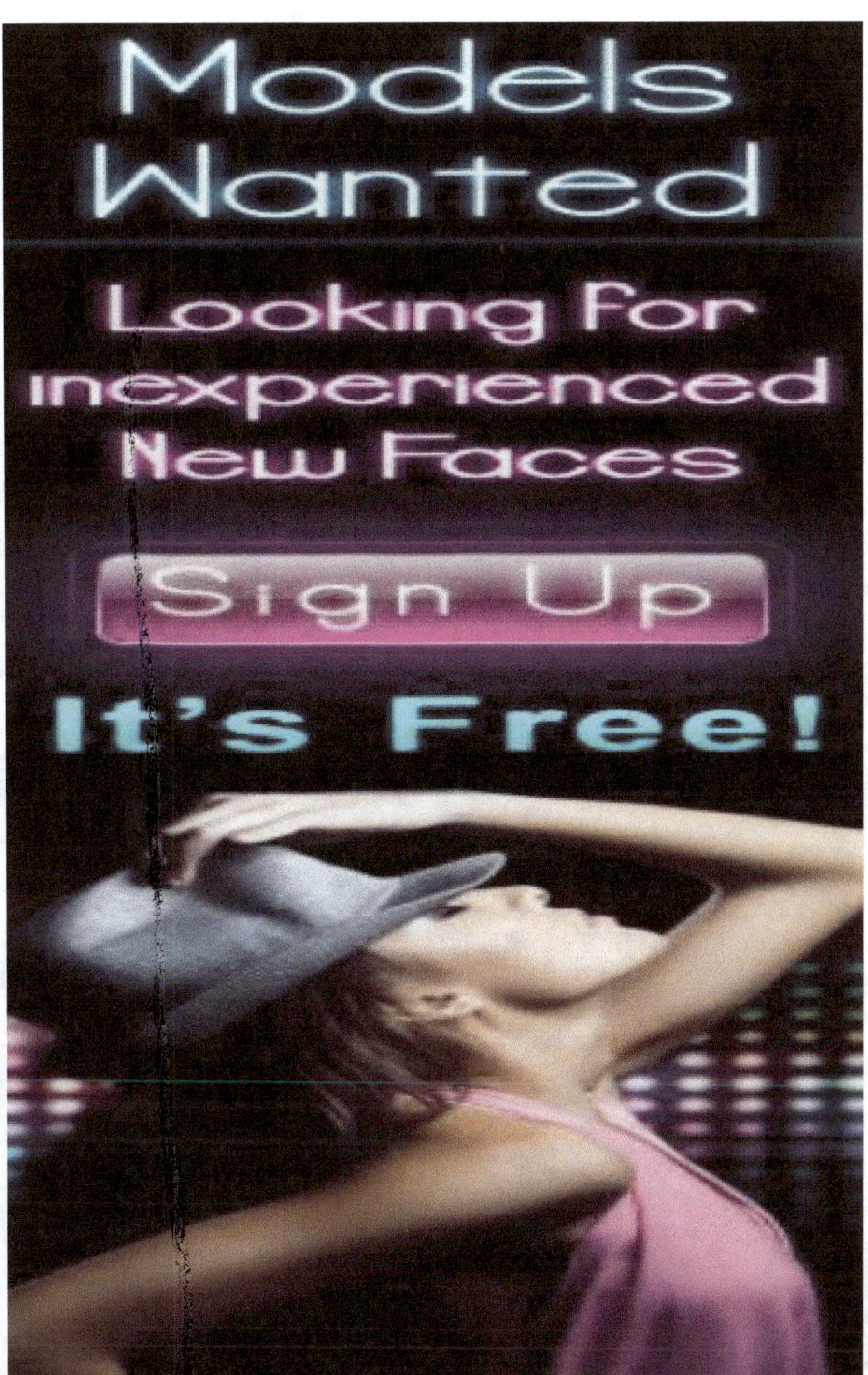

Models Wanted
Looking for inexperienced New Faces
Sign Up
It's Free!

Fit Style
ARE YOU THE NEXT
FITSTYLE AD
SPACE
MODEL?
GET YOUR PHOTO AND
FITSTYLESPACE PROFILE SEEN
WWW.CAFEPRESS.COM/FPLA

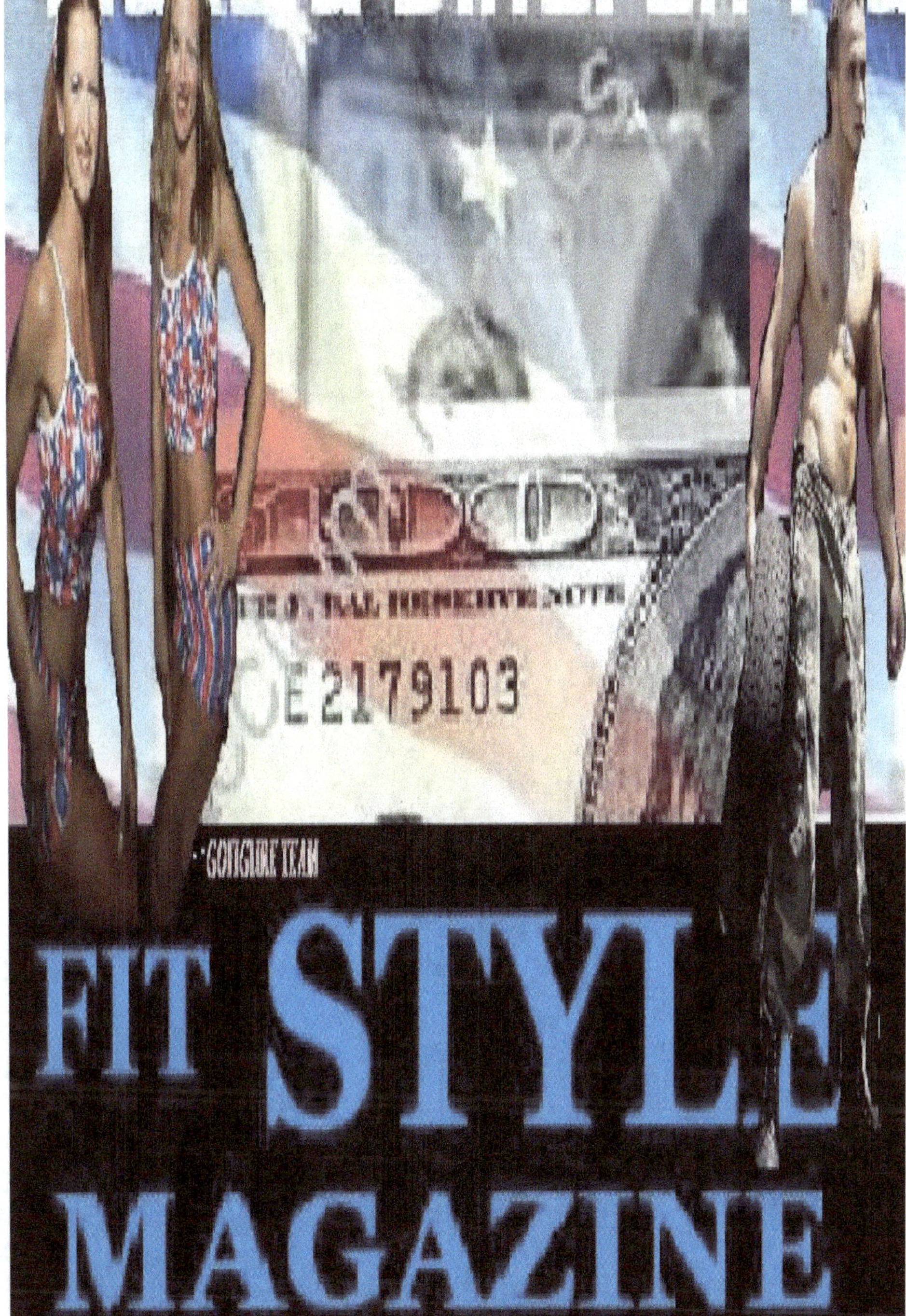
GOFIGURE TEAM
E 2179103
FIT STYLE
MAGAZINE
WWW.MYSPACE.COM/GOFIGURETEAM
DONATE A $100 OR MORE GET FREE AD
WWW.FITPROLIFESTYLE.WEBS.COM
SUPPORT THE VETERANS
JOIN TO BE AN ALL AMERICAN

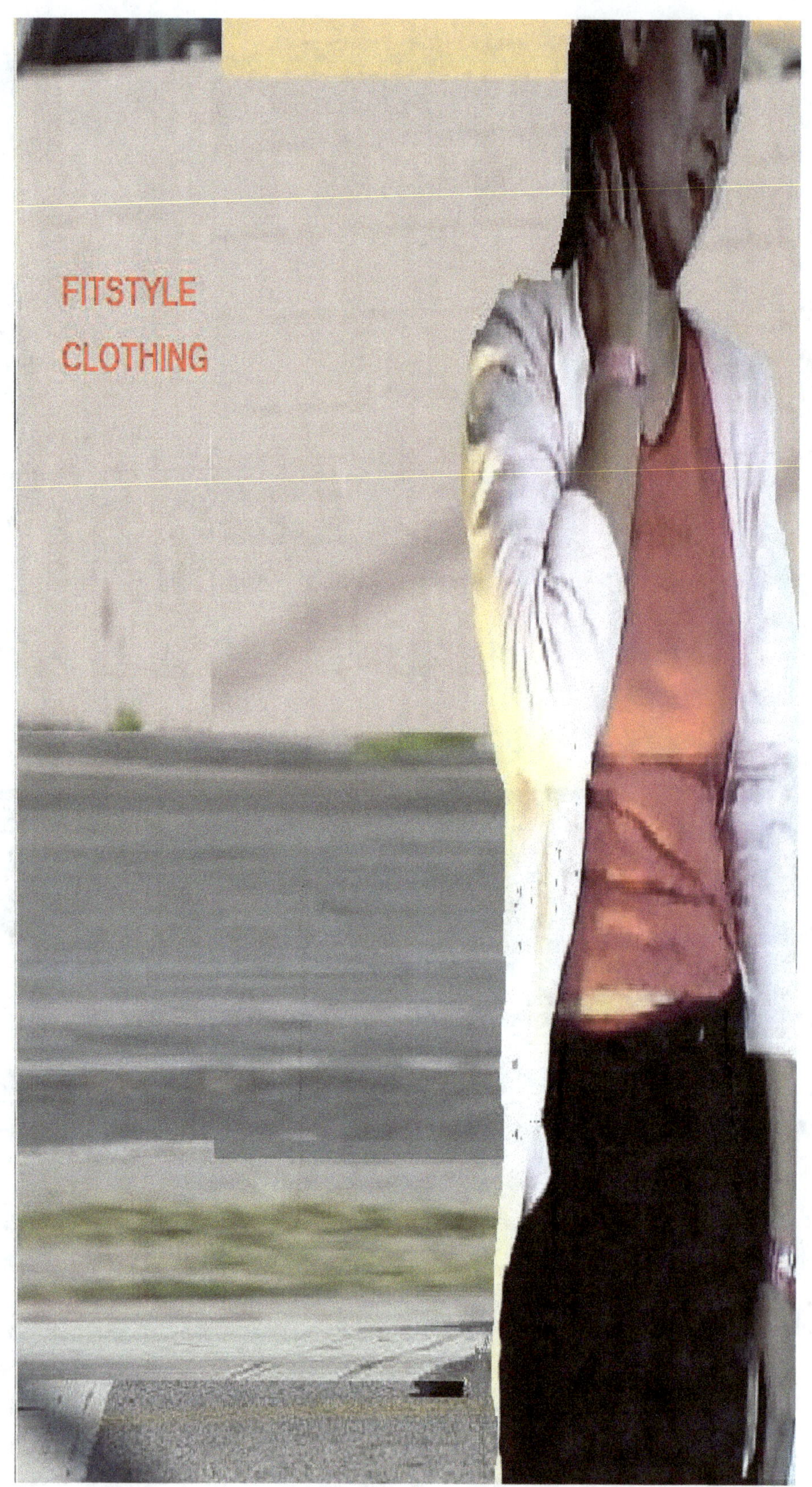

FITSTYLE
CLOTHING

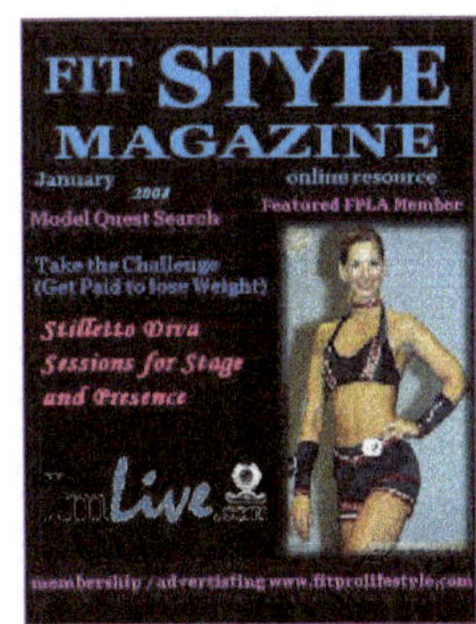
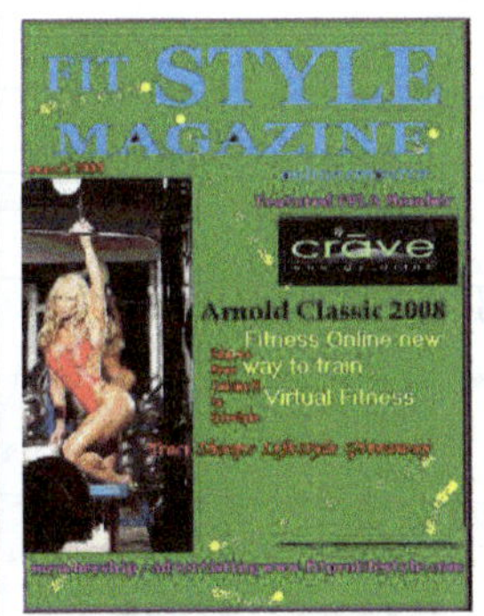
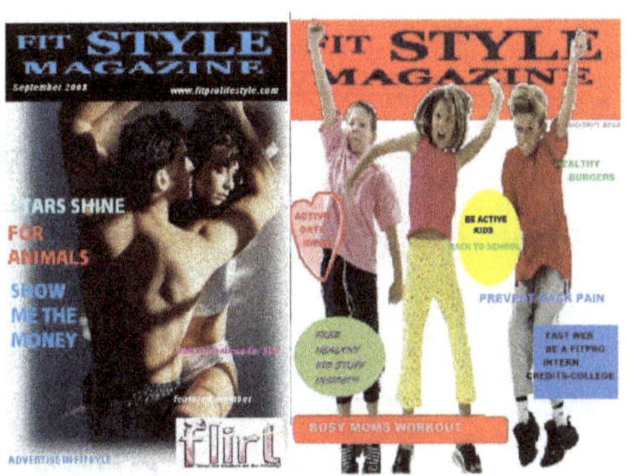

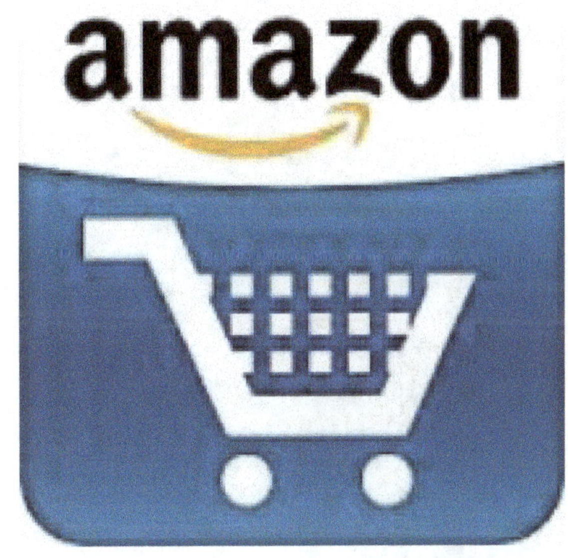

amazon

FITSTYLE FASHION ….TRENDY
Brought to you by Fitstyle Shop Style   http://www.shopstyle.com/shop/jenlclose

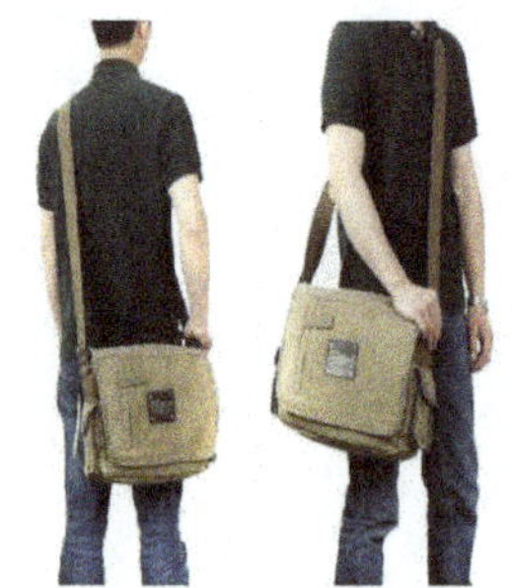

MESSENGER BAG

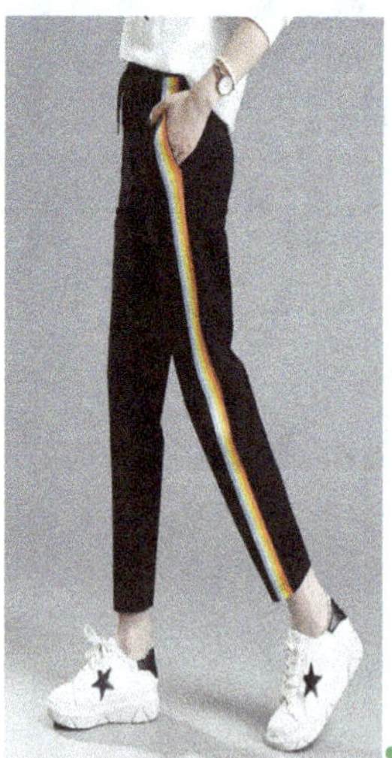

Striped Jogger Pants

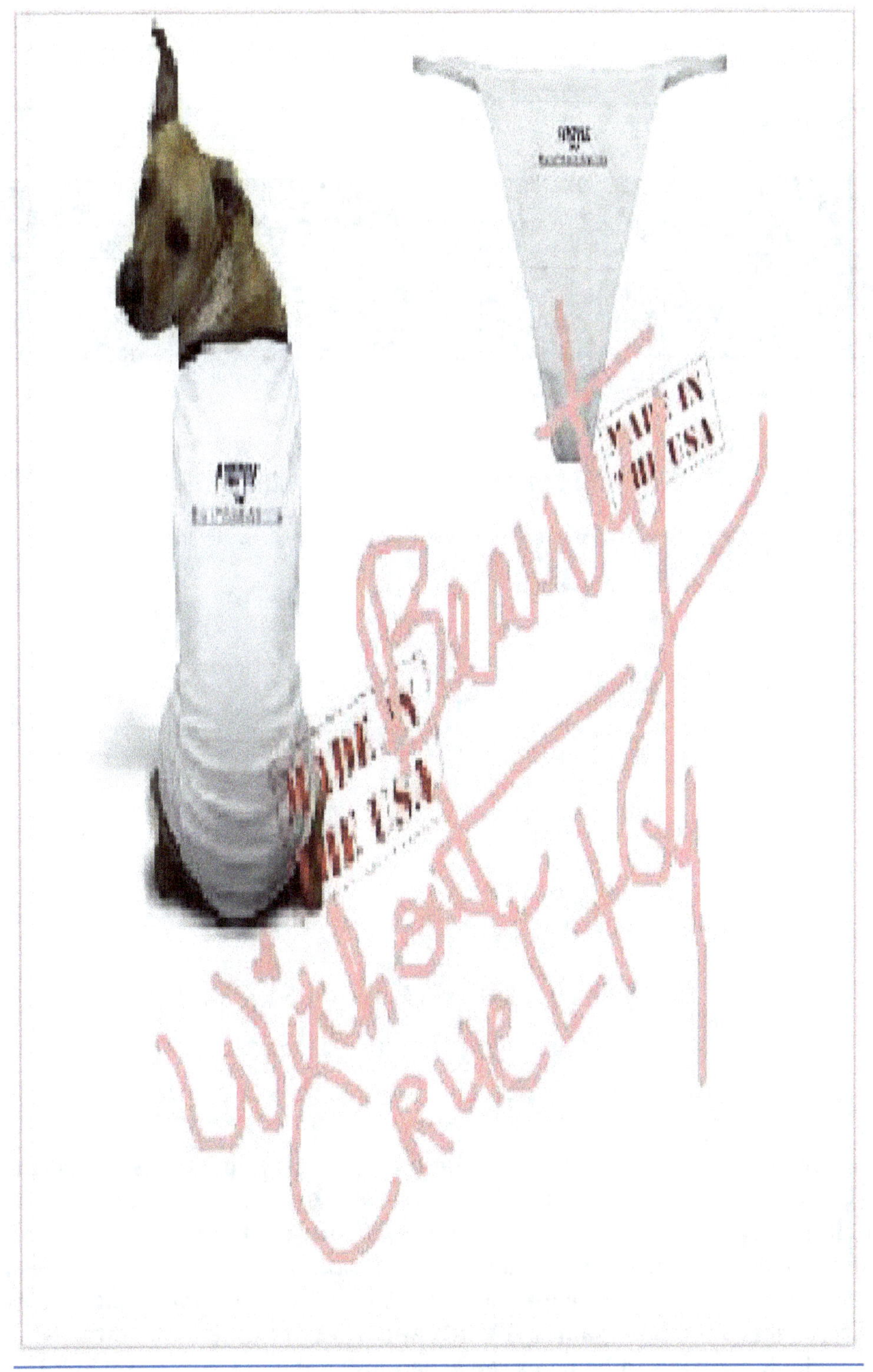

Help us by buying or donating

GIVE BACK BUY SHOPPING

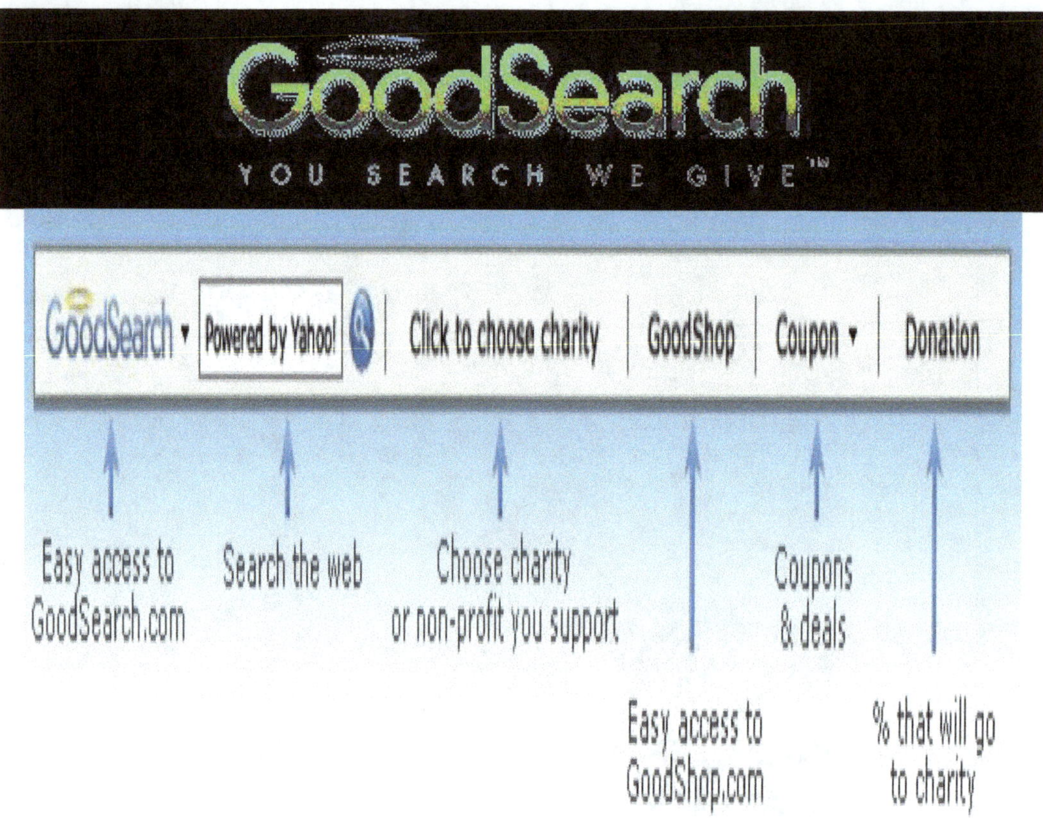

GET INVOLVED WITH GOODSEARCH

….ABCNEWS

GOODSEARCH AND GET REWARDED

If you have any concerns about how to get in on the latest home types of making extra money this is one resource that is sure to be not only fun but rewarding.   To include you are helping support without any money out of your pocket our association.   And it earns you rewards.   We are excited to also let you know that Good search has added simple easy ways for you to join with your yahoo email or Facebook and even Google profile.   The search includes games, TV ads and a way to dine with rewards.   Many times people look for ways to help get rewarded and get good karma by helping others who are presenting with their projects a way to help them and others for memberships and donations.

There are tons of ways to do this.

Fitness Professional Lifestyle Association has been researching in the latest online types of ways to make extra money for the summer or even if you have fell in hard times or health issues.   Some of them can be not as seem and they won't make you rich, but give you extra money in case you fall short or want to save up for something that you

want.   The great thing is you can earn great rewards and even CASH.   We have provided some of those here for you to check out that our members and volunteers have also checked out.

DOWNLOAD OUR NEW TOOLBAR OR MAKE US YOUR HOME PAGE

WITH EACH SEARCH YOU DO THEY WILL GIVE BACK

TO GET STARTED DOWNLOAD SAFE AND SECURE

AT   WWW.GOODSEARCH.COM/?CHARITYID=884657

EXTRA INCOME FOR SUMMER

INBOX DOLLARS- THIS IS AN OKAY SYSTEM YOU CAN TAKE SURVEY GET PAID MAIL AND GAMES WHICH JUST FOR SIGNING UP YOU GET $5

BIG BUDGET SURVEYS AND POLLS- Enter and setup through inbox and receive a $1500 sweepstakes entry plus ways to earn through the paid accounts and rewards. Plus faster with toolbar.

GLOBAL TEST MARKET- This is a way to answer questions based on client researching on products and services it sometimes requires some rejections but you will get something for at least taking the time.

ABOUT FACE- This is a mystery shopping website that never charges you and sends you job opportunities in your area or nearby to shop there with a payment and refund. You just if you see something you want to take contact the email that is registered...go to the shop do the instruction and submit the report.   But it isn't always high pay.

VINDALE-   This company has been rated that they pay every two weeks and it needs patience based on one member stating when lost work did this was dealing with rejections at first but now receiving payments every two weeks at even as much as $150 or more.

SWATCASH- This site pays you by cash or swatting it out for items or PayPal payment.   It pays on the 15th of every month.

EPOLLSURVEYS.COM- Express you with this site and earn points for cash and prizes.

MYSURVEY- This is one of the oldest survey companies.

OPINIONWOLD- This got a five star rating from members that sends you surveys and lets you even cash out at the end of the week.

CONSUMER VILLAGE- Great for FPLA members that focus on groups and offer ways to use for clients or seminars where they have discussion groups.
To learn more about others and share your opinion becomes a FPLA member today or sponsor.

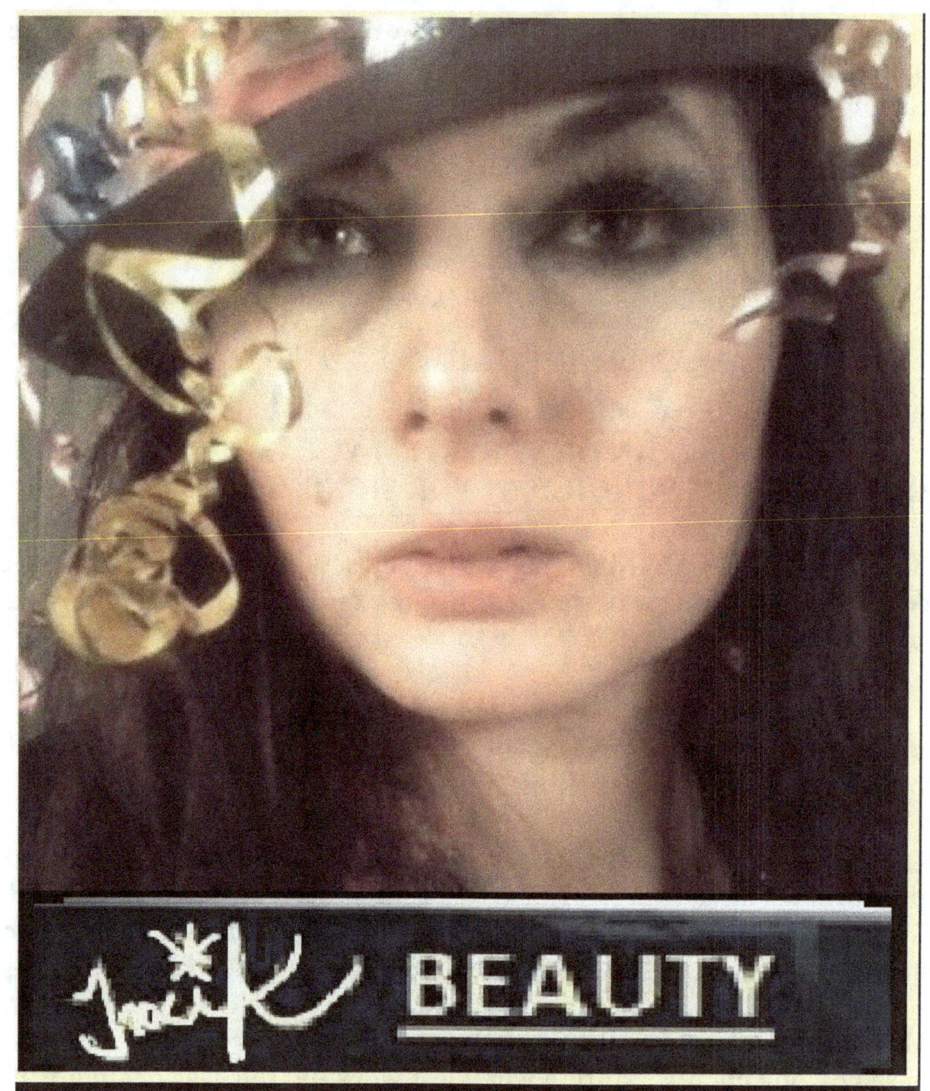

GET FREE SAMPLES, ADVICE, TIPS START YOUR PROFILE

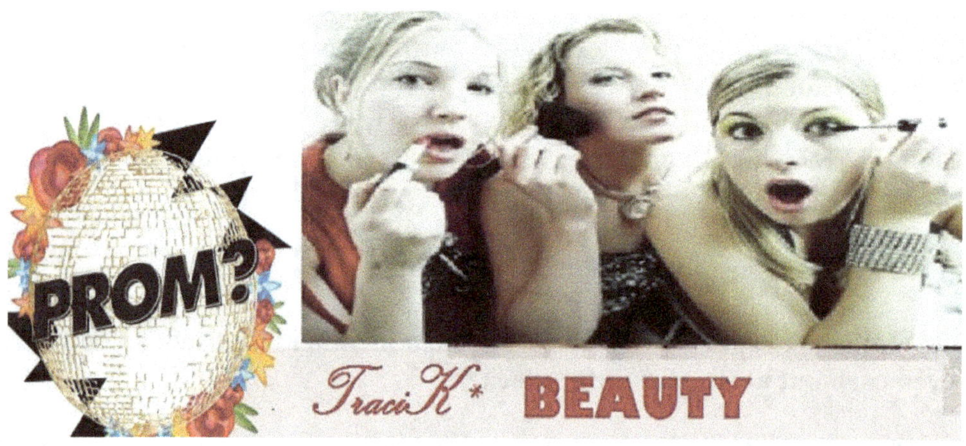

5 ways to

SEXY FLAT ABS

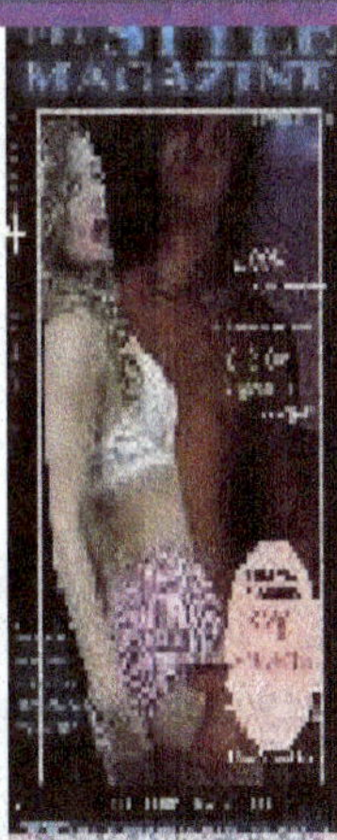

ORDER TODAY

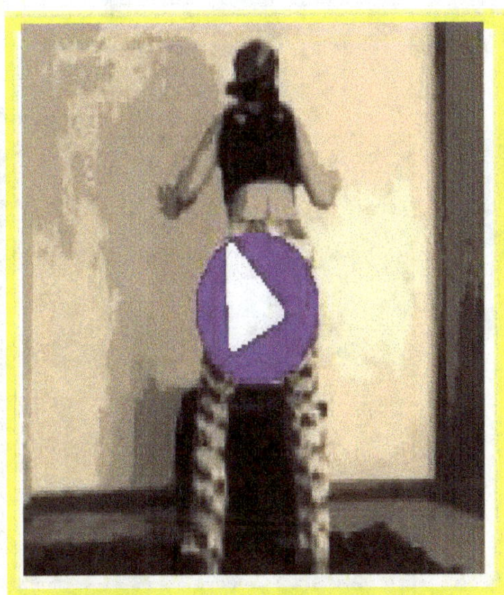

trendiest training videos

reality show boot camp

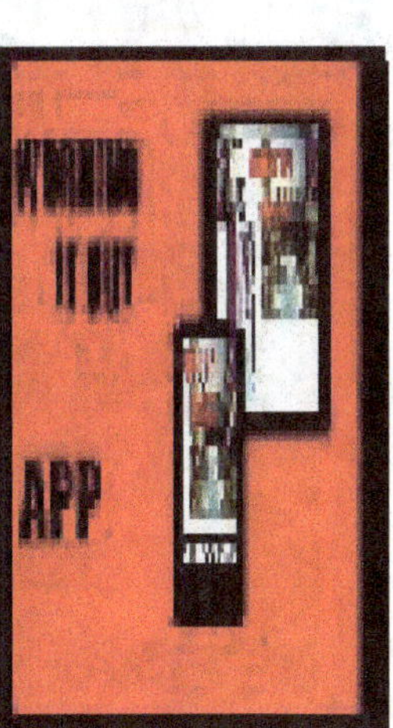

new mobile app

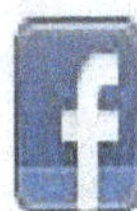

Facebook

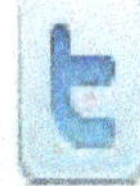

Twitter

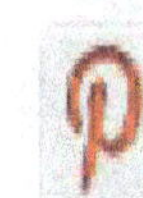

Pinterest

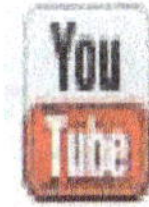

YouTube

connect to Fitstylemag

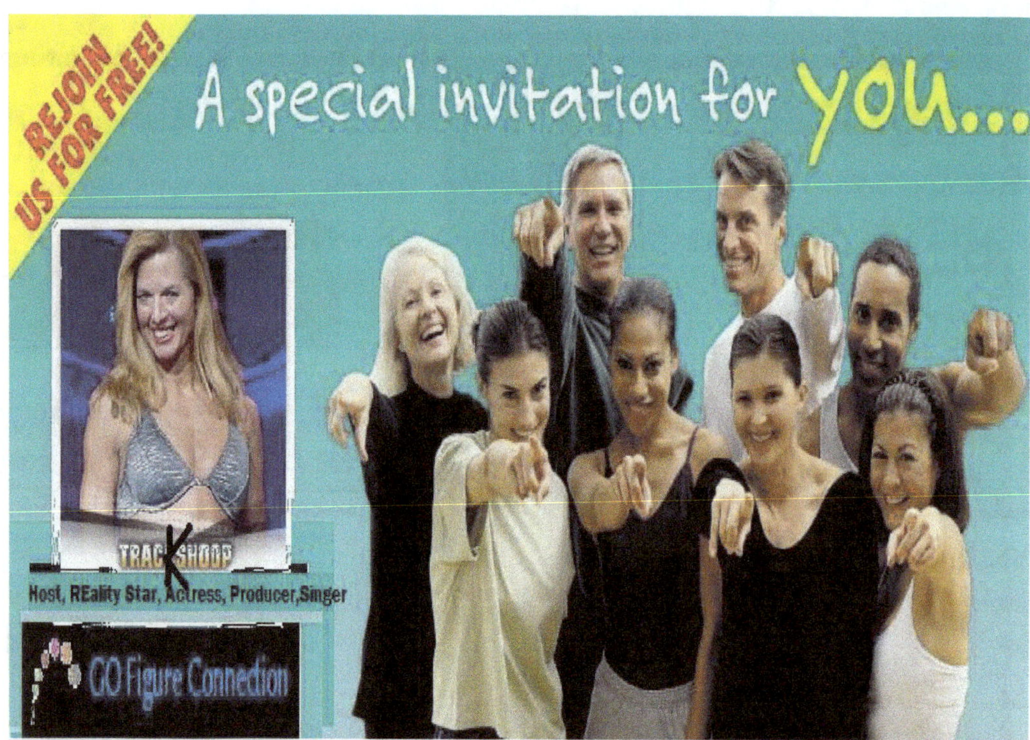

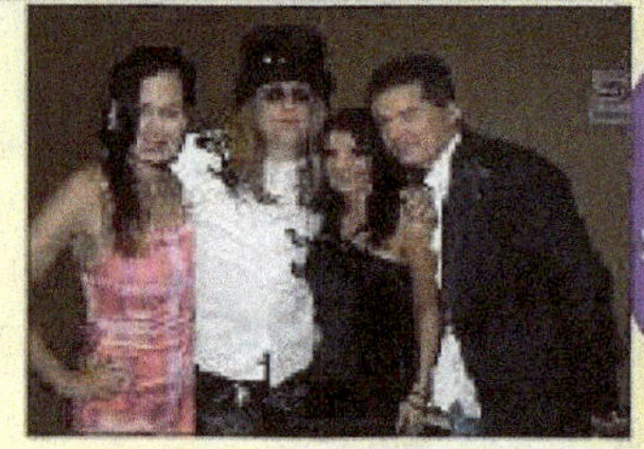

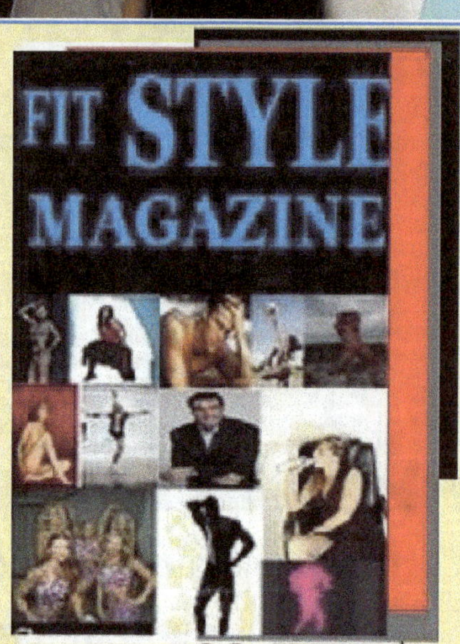

EVERY ISSUE:
FITNESS PROFESSIONALS
LIFESTYLE TIPS
INTERVIEWS *CELEBS
NEVER SEEN PHOTOS
FITSTYLE SHOOTOUTS
SPECIAL OFFERS FOR
MEMBERS ONLY

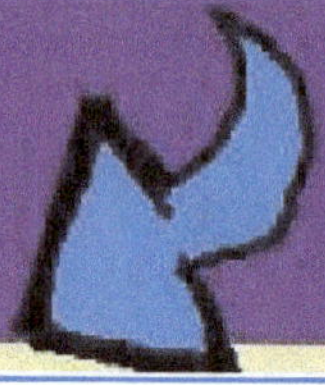

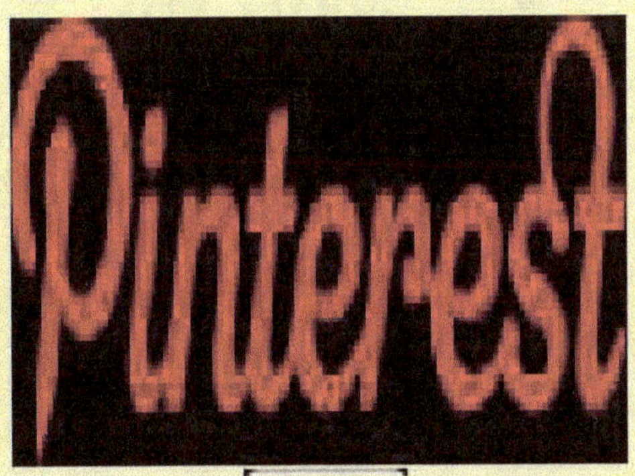

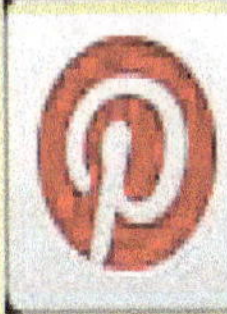

Follow me on *Pinterest*

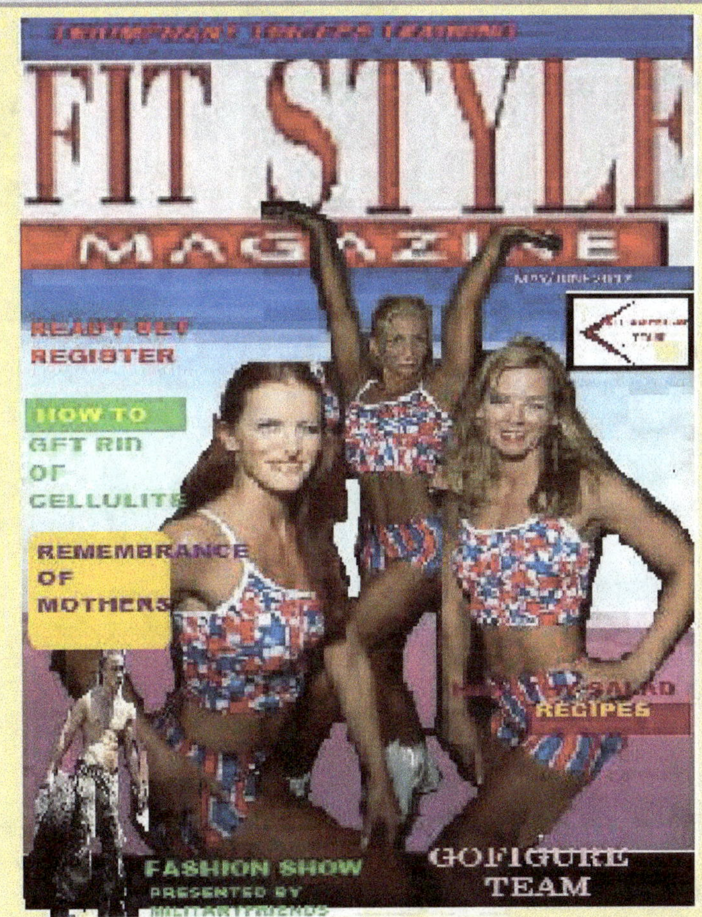

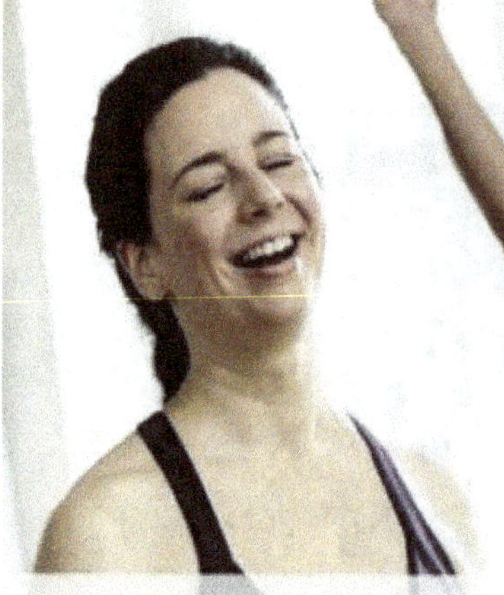

KRISTIN W. LOST 114 POUNDS, WON $4,000!

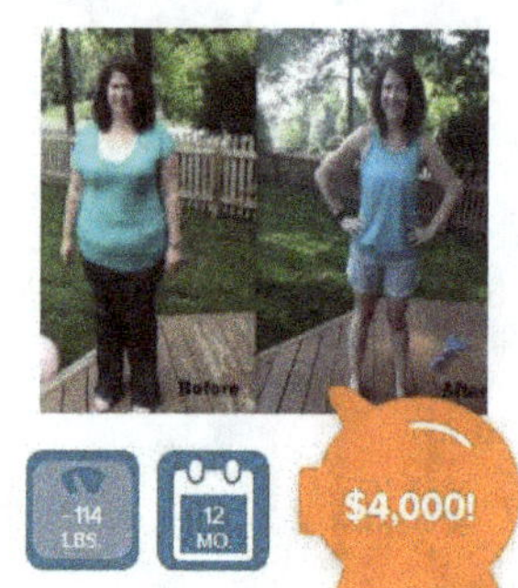

JENNIFER D. LOST 102 POUNDS, WON $4,181!

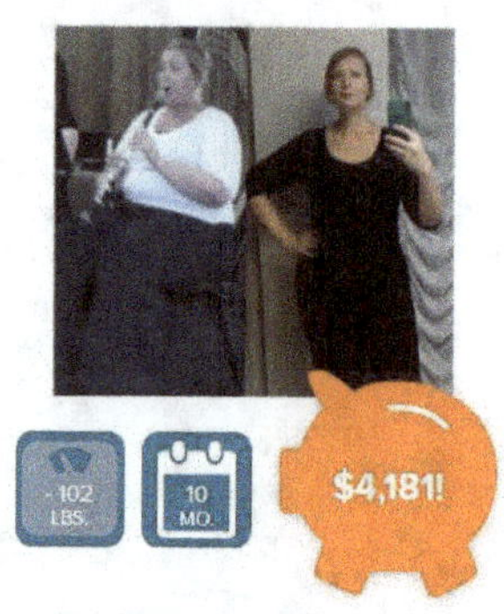

GLENN S. LOST 102 POUNDS, WON $1,383!

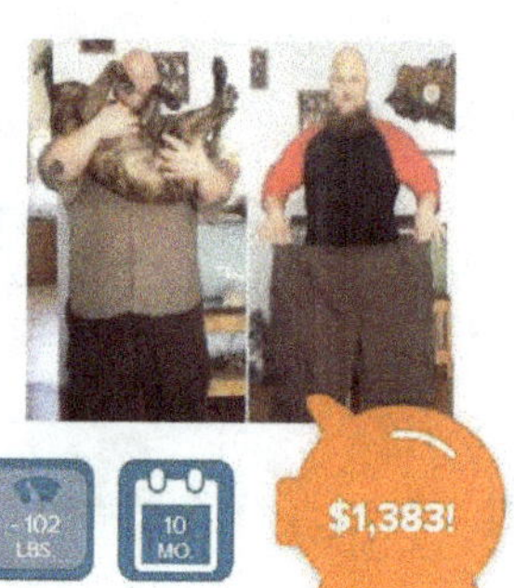

How it Works

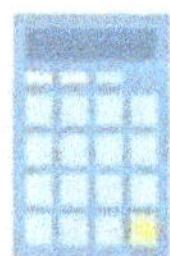

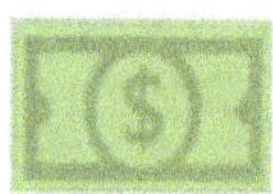

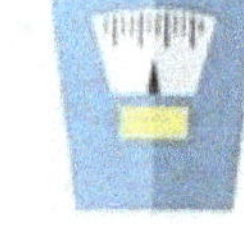

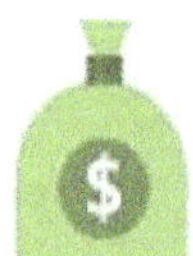

1) Calculate Your Prize

Use our calculator to enter your goal and calculate your winnings.

2) Make Your Bet

Increase your winnings by adjusting your goal weight, how much you contribute, and the time you expect it to take! Find a prize you like and make your wager!

3) Lose the Weight

Stay on track throughout the contest with weekly weigh-ins and support from other contestants.

4) Win Money!

Meet your goal and win your prize! It's that simple!

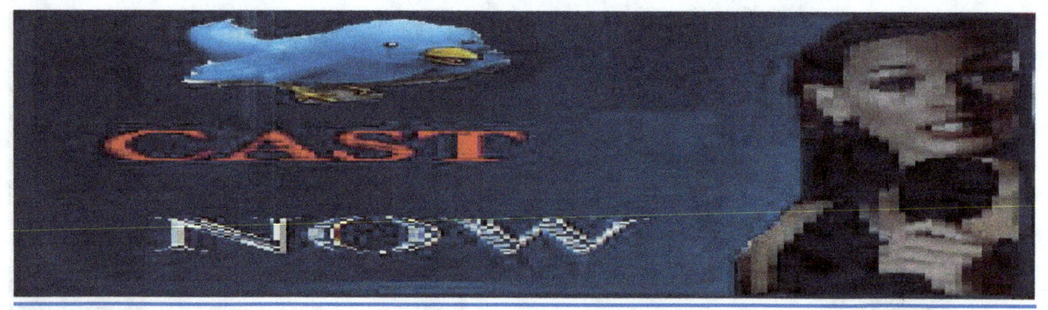

YOUR TURN FITSTYLE BEAUTY AWARDS NOMINATE YOUR OWN

BEST NAIL SALON

BEST HAIR SALON

BEST MAKEUP ARTIST

BEST FASHION SHOW

FAVORITE LIP GLOSS

FAVORITE MASCARA

FAVORITE EYE SHADOW

BEST HAIR STYLIST PRODUCT

BEST CLOTHING STORE

BEST FITNESS DESIGNER

BEST GYM TO MEET PEOPLE

HEALTHIEST NITECLUB

BEST PROTEIN POWDER

BEST ENERGY PRODUCT

BEST WEIGHT LOSS PRODUCT

FAVORITE STYLIST

FAVORITE TRAINER

HEALTHIEST FRIENDLIEST PLACE TO EAT

FITSTYLE FEMALE OF THE YEAR

FITSTYLE MALE OF THE YEAR

BEST HAIRSPRAY

BEST NAIL PRODUCT

FAVORITE SHAMPOO

FAVORITE CONDITIONER

BEST SKIN PRODUCT FOR WRINKLES

BEST SKIN PRODUCT FOR ADULT ACNE

BEST SHOES TO RUN ON TRAILS

BEST SHOES FOR DANCING

BEST SHOES FOR WEIGHT TRAINING

BEST STAGE JEWELRY DESIGNER

BEST MASSAGE THERAPIST

BEST MOTIVATIONAL ALBUM OF THE YEAR

BEST MOTIVATIONAL MOVIE OF THE YEAR

FITSTYLE US ARMY OF THE YEAR

FITSTYLY US NAVY OF THE YEAR

FITSTYLE US AIR FORCE OF THE YEAR

FITSTYLE US MARINE OF THE YEAR

YOUR FAVORITE FITSTYLE COVER OF THE YEAR

YOUR ADDED NOMINATION:

HAVE A SUCCESS STORY SET UP YOUR PROFILE
WWW.FITPROLIFESTYLE.WEBS.COM TELL YOUR STORY

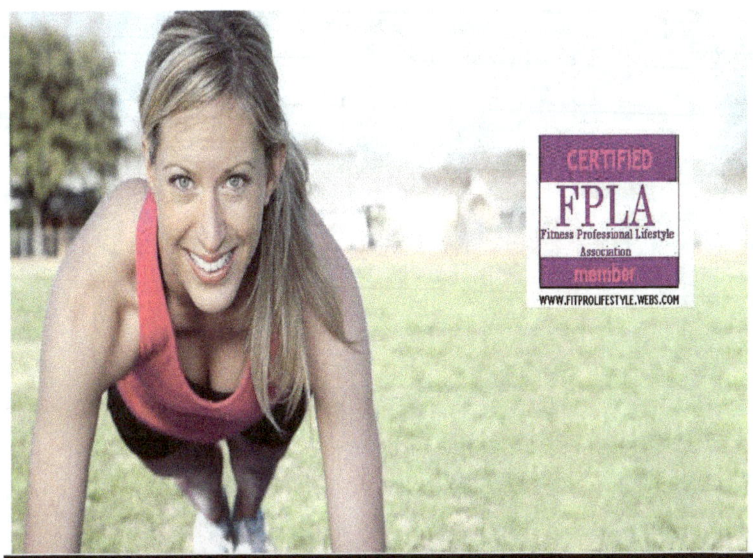

CERTIFIED
FPLA
Fitness Professional Lifestyle
Association
member
WWW.FITPROLIFESTYLE.WEBS.COM

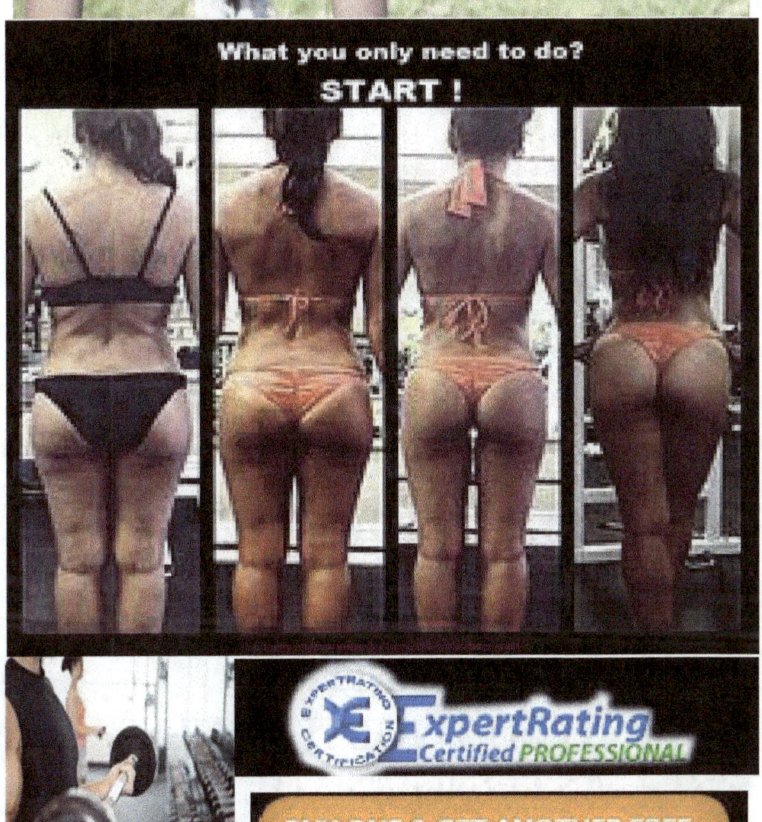

What you only need to do?
START !
ExpertRating
Certified PROFESSIONAL
BUY ONE & GET ANOTHER FREE

HAPPY MOTHERS DAY

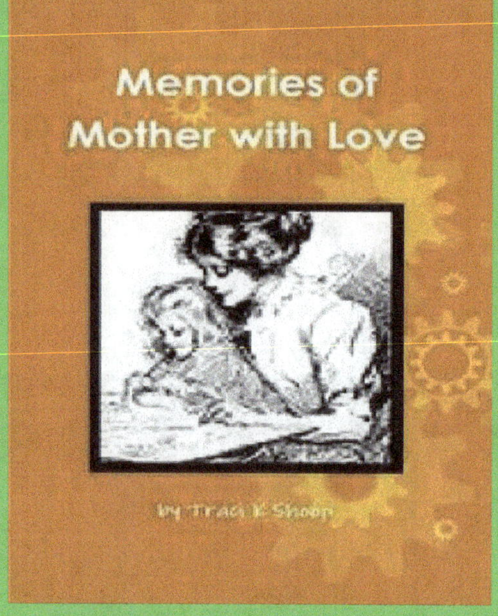

A STRONG
FRIENDSHIP DOESN'T
NEED DAILY
CONVERSATION,
DOESN'T ALWAYS
NEED TOGETHERNESS,
AS LONG AS THE
RELATIONSHIP LIVES
IN THE HEART,
TRUE FRIENDS
WILL NEVER PART...

ABOUT IT.
First come first serve..do you want   to have youR book showcaseD at one of the top Expos in MAY…

you can with us only 8-10 authors will be chosen for the shelf case..get scene by over 60,000 publishers, agent and book lovers,…and art exhibit for your book..   To get a chance to be part of this go to click on EXPO.. And register.. Must send at least two copies to be display..

IF YOU DON'T MAKE IT THIS TIME THERE WILL BE MORE AND WE ALSO PICK UP TO 5 BOOKS TO PROMOTE ON OUR CAROSELL
GOOD LUCK.
EVENT IS AT THE END OF MAY

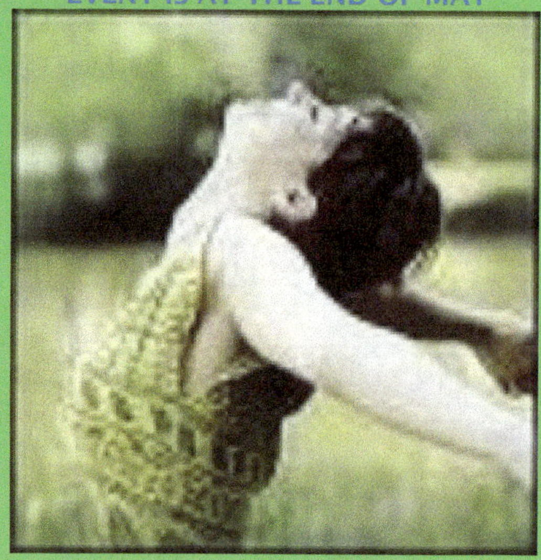

BECOME FPLA MEMBER TODAY AND HELP…

WWW.VOLUNTEERMATCH.COM
SPONSORS WELCOMED FOR THE MODEL SEARCH

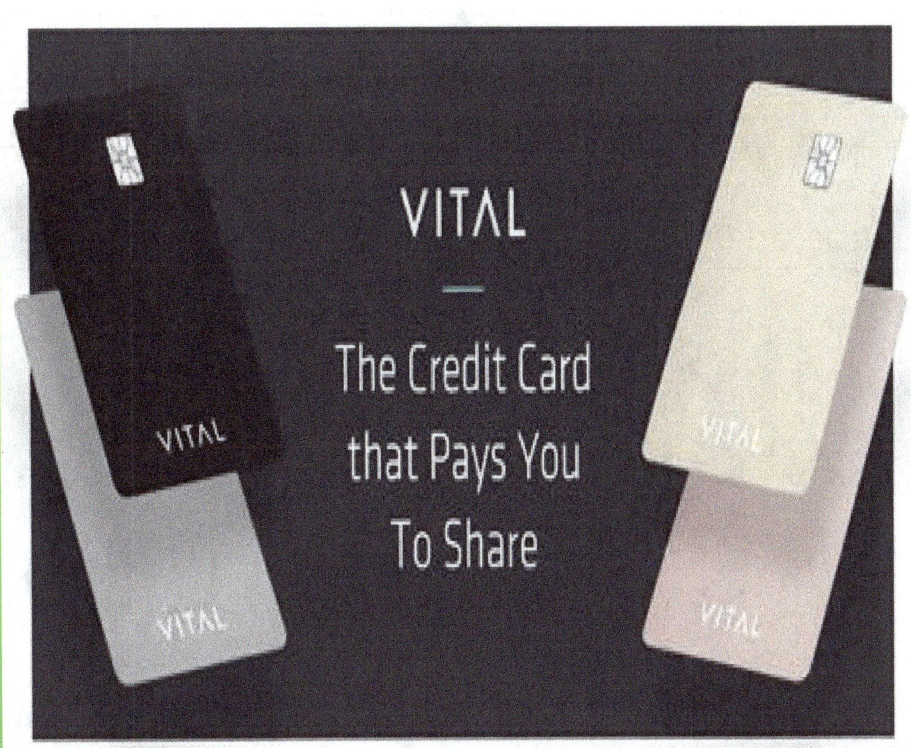

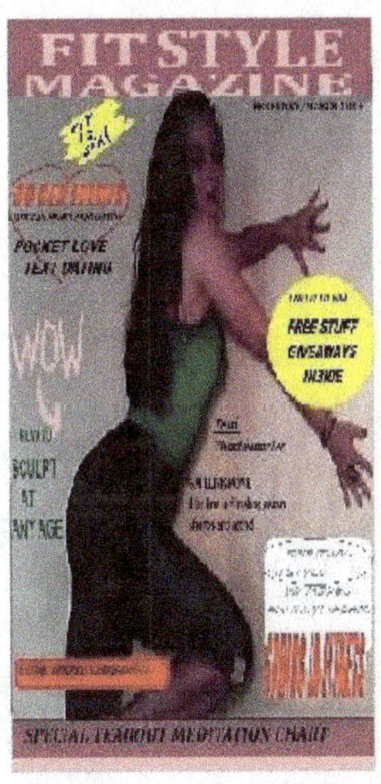

GET FREE UPGRADE
FITSTYLE MAGAZINE

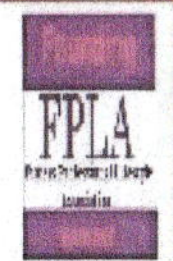

SPONSOR
AN AD SUPPORT
WOMEN, ATHLETES,
VETERANS,
ADVERTISE TO CELEBS.

FITNESS PROS
BECOME A MEMBER
OF FPLA ......

COUPON GOOD FOR ONE ISSUE

AD RUNS FOR EXTRA MONTH
FOR NEW CLIENTS ONLY

SHOWCASE YOUR SERVICE OR PRODUCT

COULD BE TAX DEDUCTIBLE

ADVERTISE YOUR COMPANY

UPLOAD ONLINE WWW.FITPROLIFESTYLE.WEBS.COM

CONTACT AT FITSTYLEMAG@AOL.COM

WWW.INSTAGRAM.COM/FITSTYLEMAGAZINE * TWITTER @FITSTYLEMAG

POWERED BY
WEBS

FIT BEACH BODY CONTEST WWW.FACEBOOK.COM/FITSTYLEMAGAZINE

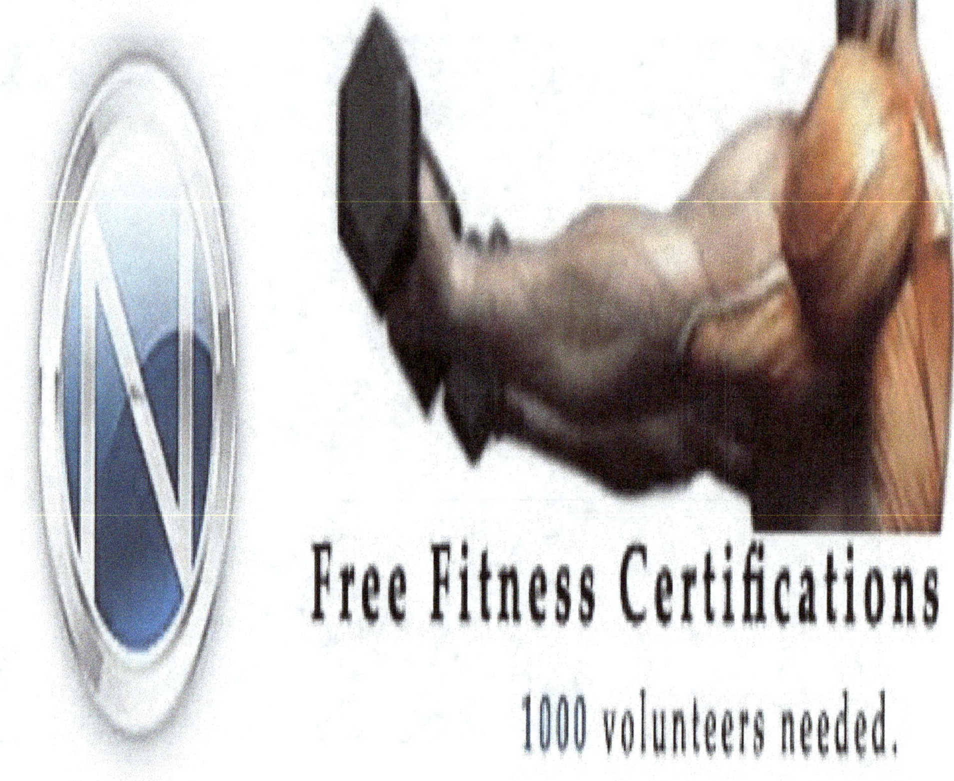

Send an online gift subscription of FitStyle Free to someone you care about:
Your Name________________ email:________________
Address____
Gift Name ______________email:________________
Address____
Gift Name______________ email________________
Address____
Cut this out and mail it to   5440 Dunmore Dr. suite 118 Dayton,Ohio45459
Attn: Gift of Online FitStyle Magazine with note.

Support Your Troops Morale sends this issue to a soldier friend that is away …with a KISS…
Send a check or money order of $25 and we will send an issue to them with a note from you.   If you have someone in mind please let us know below.
To pay by credit card you can also send this by visiting www.lulu.com/fitstylemagazine.

To send a gift of FitStyle to a soldier away and help us send magazines over…to them FREE
Send your donation to GFC Consulting 3828 harden rd. suite 118 Hope Mills NC 28348 Could be tax-deductible…visit www.fitprolifestyle.webs.com for more info.

SEE YOUR AD HERE $100   CONTACT US
GFCCONNECTION@GMAIL.COM

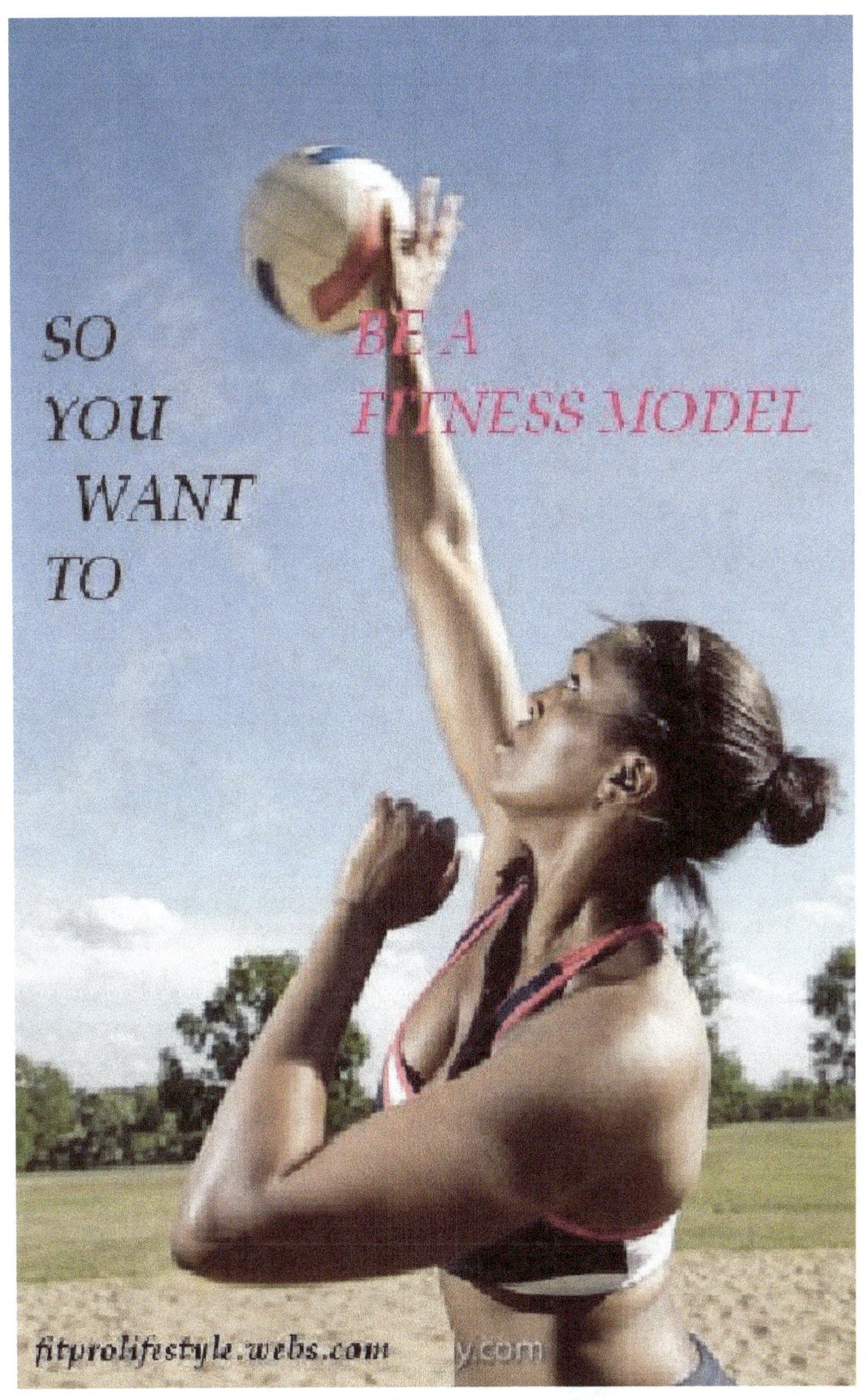

With your donation of $5 get the BOOK …2009 FitStyle Model Nina Webber
www.lulu.com/spotlight/fitstylemagazine.

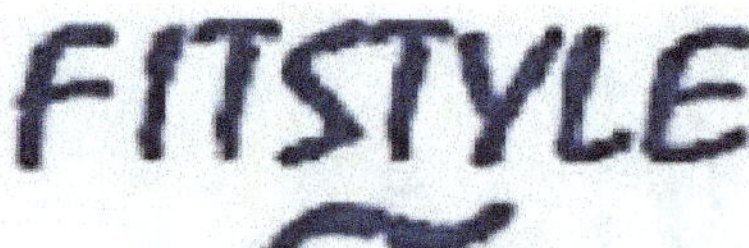

WIN A TOTE BAG

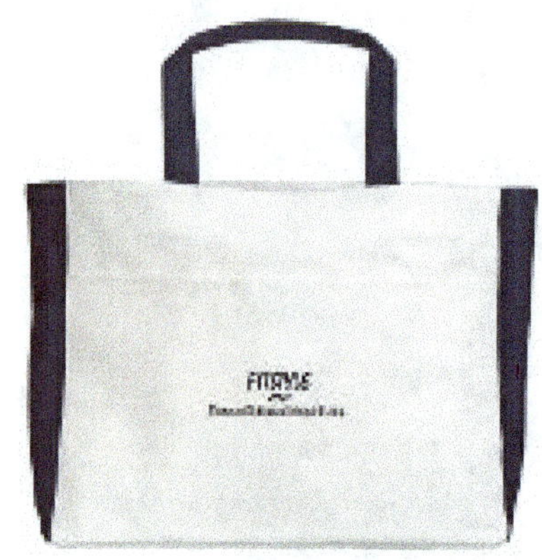

SUBMIT YOUR FITSTYLE PHOTOS ONLINE INSTAGRAM #FITSTYLEMAGAZINE
Presented by café press
Show your creative FitStyle
Contact them and ask for it....mention FitStyle and see about discounts
GET A HD CAMARA and submit your videos in our network...
www.cafepress.com/fpla

LOSING WEIGHT
WITH STYLE

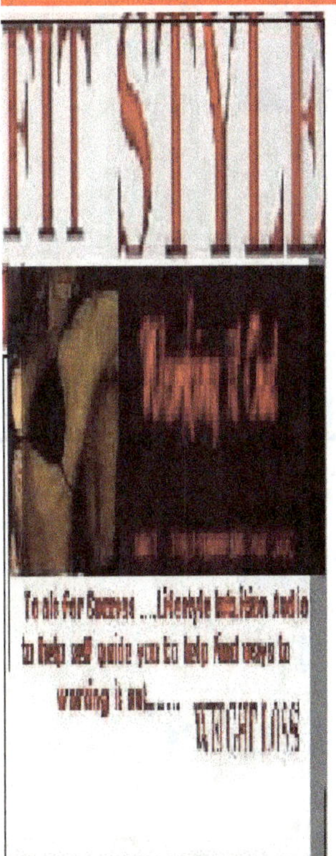

FiTStyle Recipes ......
Transform your eating habits with
delicious recipes from FiTStyle.

up to 9 different
categories and
motivational tips
and photos
-poultry
-meat
-shakes
-Sandwiches
-Seafood

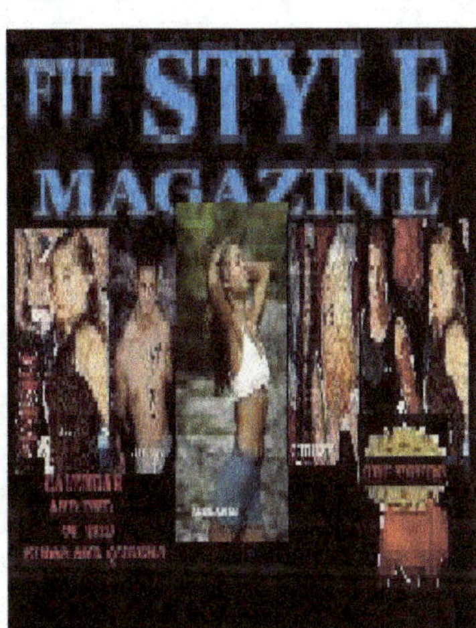

FiTSTyle CALENDAR

Get the calendar with our
had picked models who
are supporting....

melanie pitts, chrissy,Traci,John
Steinhaus and many more...visit their
profile on our online community.

**BONUS SAVE MORE WHEN YOU PURCHASE
THEM TOGETHER**

SIGN UP FOR OUR ONLINE PUBLICATION to get up to date info

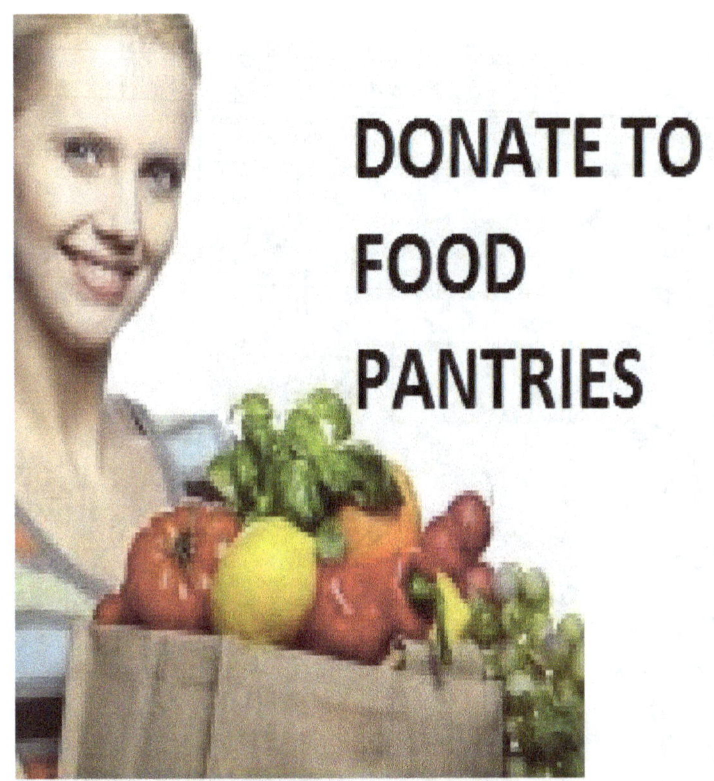

TO LOCATE YOUR FOOD
PANTRY IN YOUR CITY

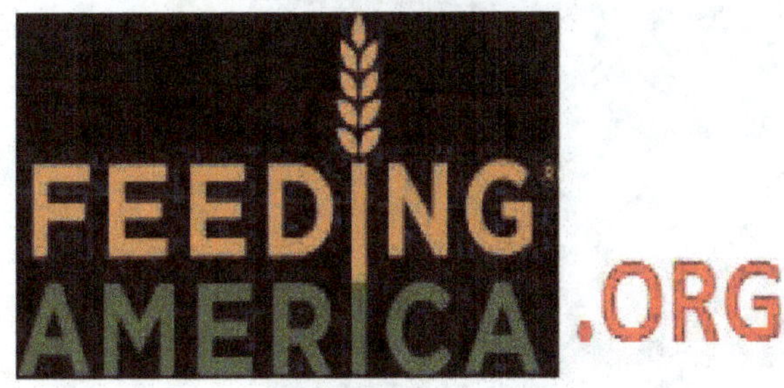

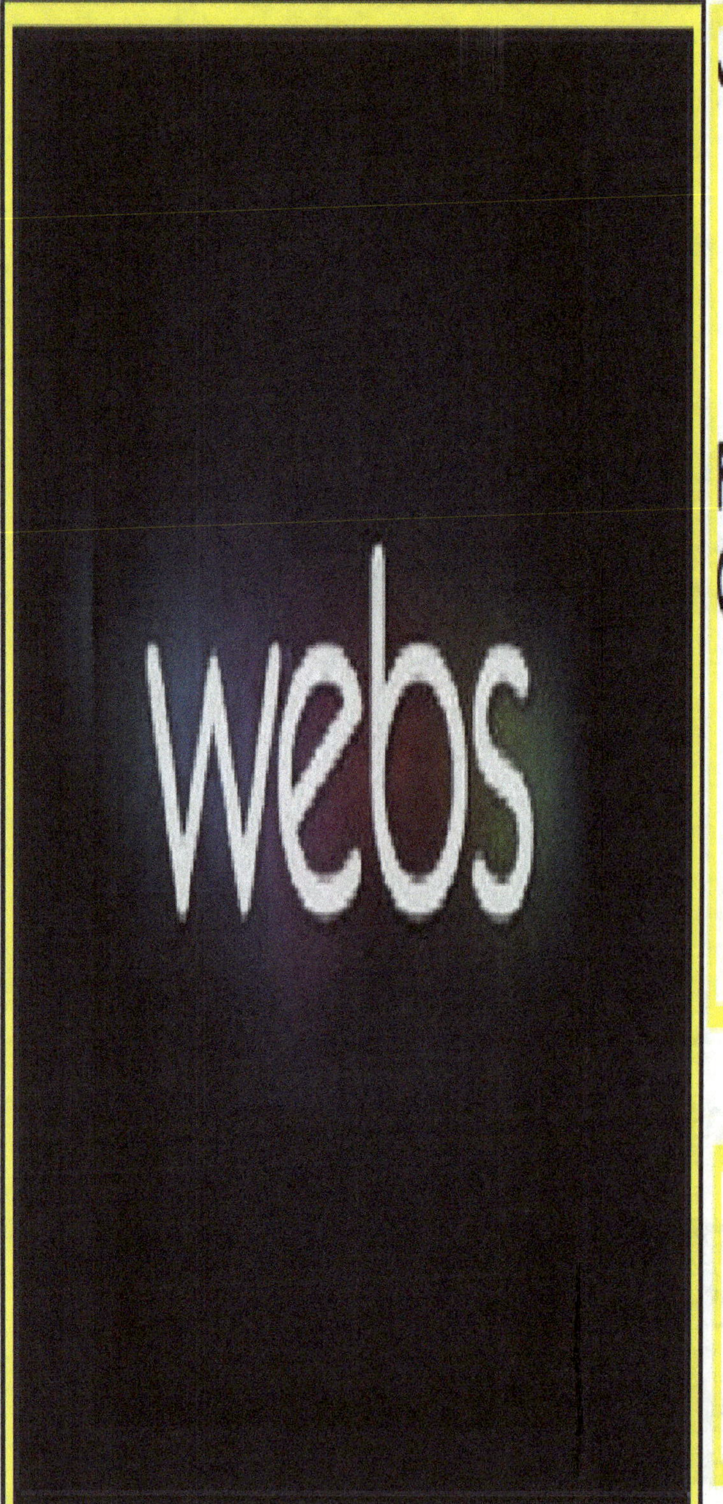

webs

JOIN

NETWORK

FREE WEBSITE
OFFICIAL FPLA

SPONSOR

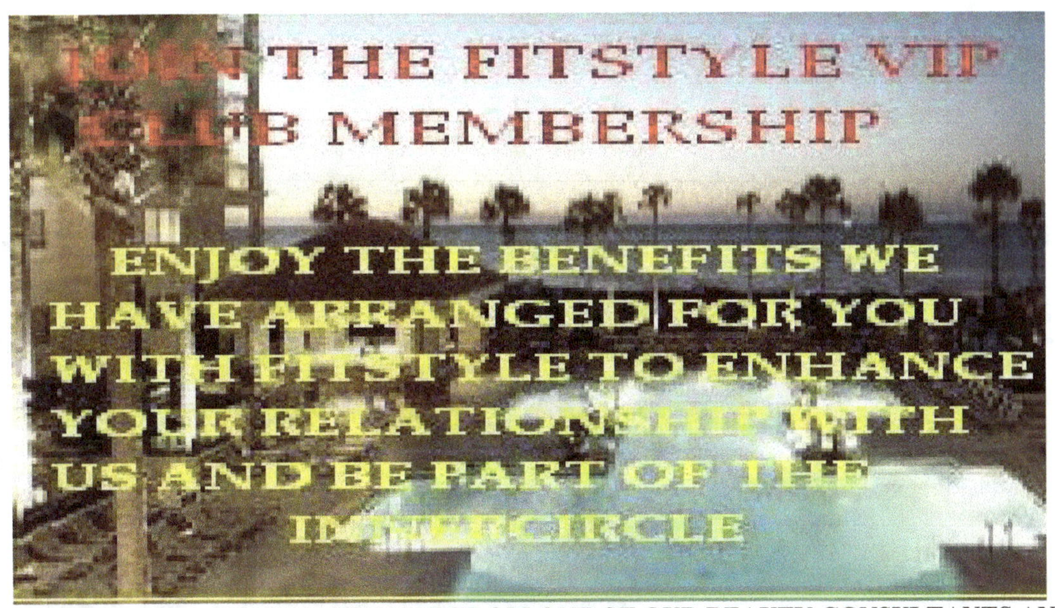

REGISTER FOR A FREE MAKEOVER FROM ONE OF OUR BEAUTY CONSULTANTS AND HELP SOMEONE DURING HARD TIMES
WE RECOMMEND THESE PRODUCTS   HELP US REVIEW THEM…
ADVERTISE HERE FOR ONLY $100 contact us online or email gofigureliveadvice@yahoo.com

WE NEED PRODUCT REVIEWS EMAIL US YOUR QUESTIONS

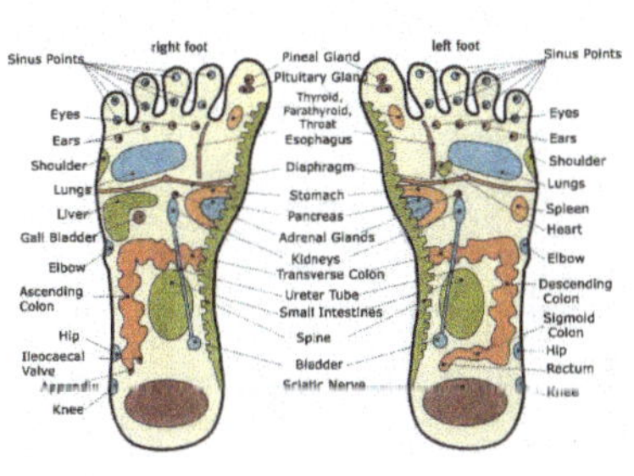

Get the tips on reflexology and where the points are….

TRUE LEMON PACKETS.
WANT FREE SAMPLES
SIGN UP AND PAY   AS A MEMBER
AND WE WILL SEND YOU

INFO ON HOW TO GET THEM….

ONE WEEK FREE PASS
TO SELF DEFENSE CLASSES

AND LEARN MARTIAL ARTS FOR HEALTH

TO GET THIS AND MUCH MORE

REGISTER BECOME A MEMBER

ADVERTISE IN OUR MARKETPLACE
CONTACT JENN
JGFCGROUP@AOL.COM

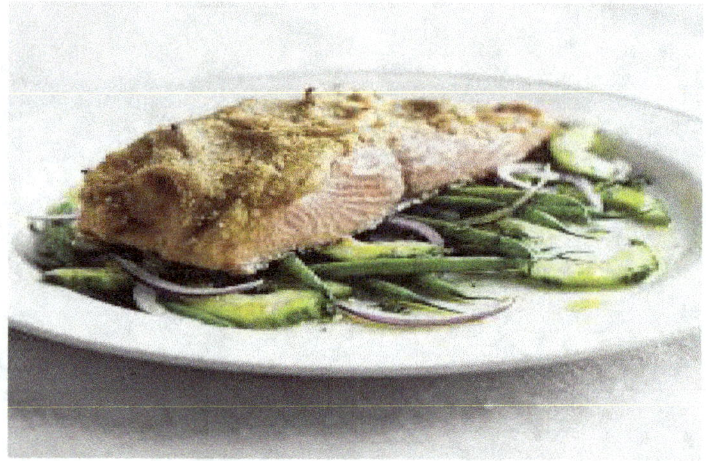

For the Dressing

1 garlic clove, finely chopped
200g natural yogurt
200ml tahini
juice of 3 lemons

For the fish

4kg boneless, skin-on salmon fillet zest and juice of 1-2 lemons

200g fresh coriander, leaves picked
120g fresh mint, leaves picked and roughly chopped
300g walnuts, dry-fried until very dark and aromatic, then coarsely chopped
2 tsp sumac
seeds from 1 pomegranate
180g hummus
1 red onion, finely chopped

150ml extra-virgin olive oil **METHOD:** Put the garlic, yogurt and tahini into a bowl with 1 tsp salt and stir to blend. Add enough lemon juice too thin to the consistency of pouring cream. Season to taste and chill.

Preheat the oven to 180C/gas mark 4 and line a baking tray with baking parchment. Roast the salmon on the tray until almost cooked through – about 15-20 minutes. Remove from oven and leave to cool to room temperature.

Meanwhile, set aside a small amount of the lemon zest, coriander and mint to decorate. Mix the walnuts, lemon juice, remaining zest and herbs, sumac and half the pomegranate seeds. Set aside.

Put the salmon on a serving platter and pour the dressing over. Spread over the hummus, then the walnut mixture. Scatter over the reserved herbs, lemon zest and pomegranate seeds, and drizzle over as much oil as you like. Serve.

LEARN THE DIFFERENCE

FASHION MODELS

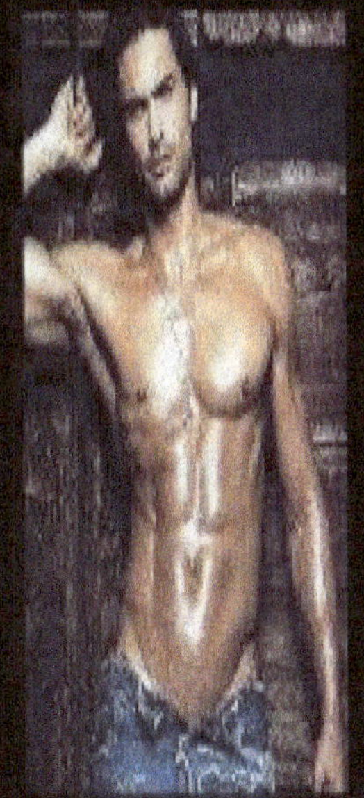

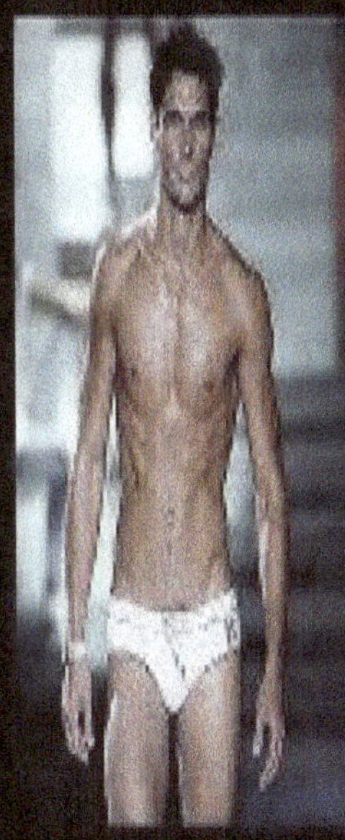

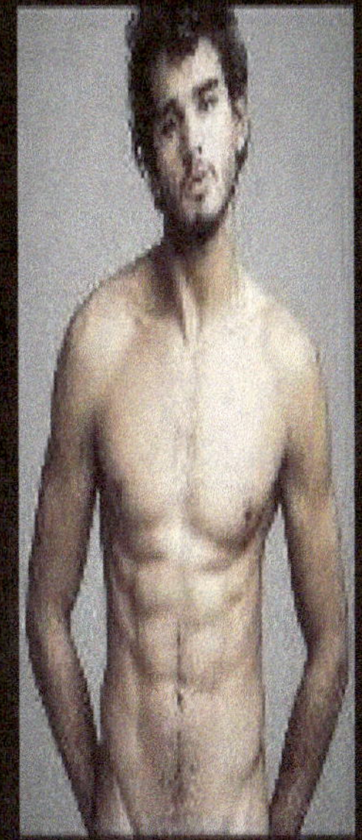

MARCUS SCHENCENBERG · DAVID GANDY · MARLON TEIXEIRA

FITNESS MODELS

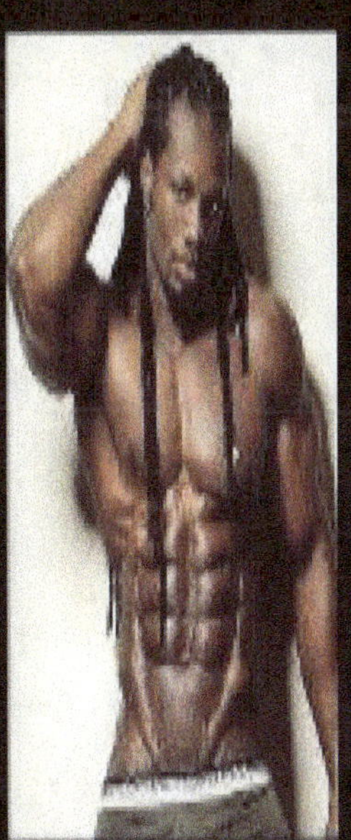

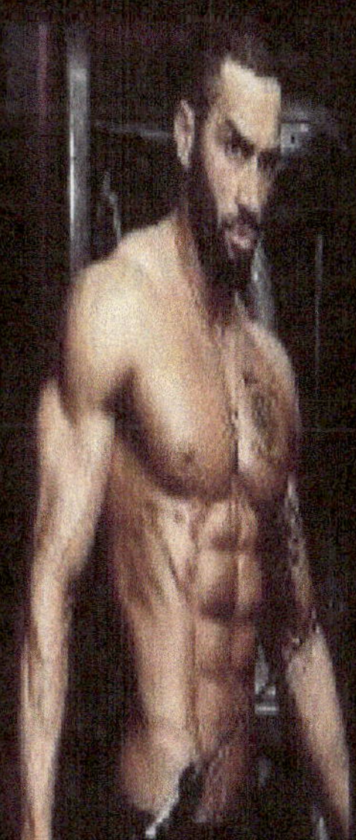

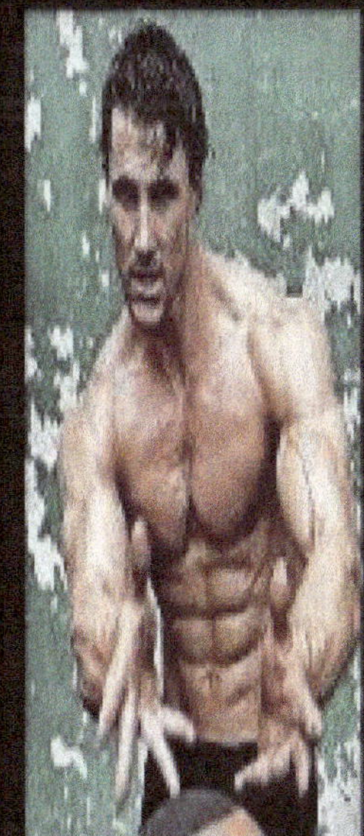

ULISSES WILLIAMS · LAZAR ANGELOV · GREG PLITT

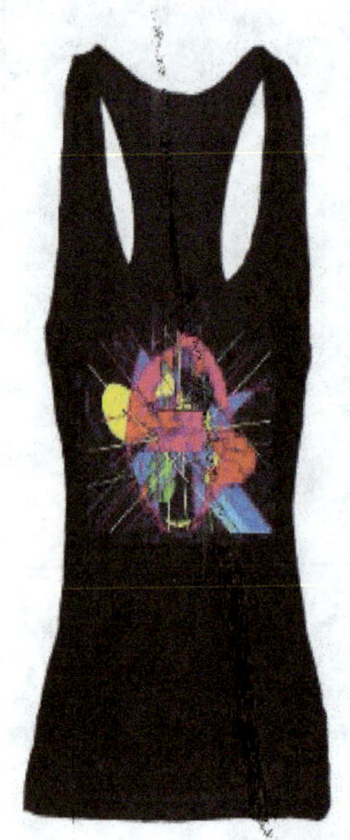

FITSTYLE ZUMBA WEAR BY TRACI K

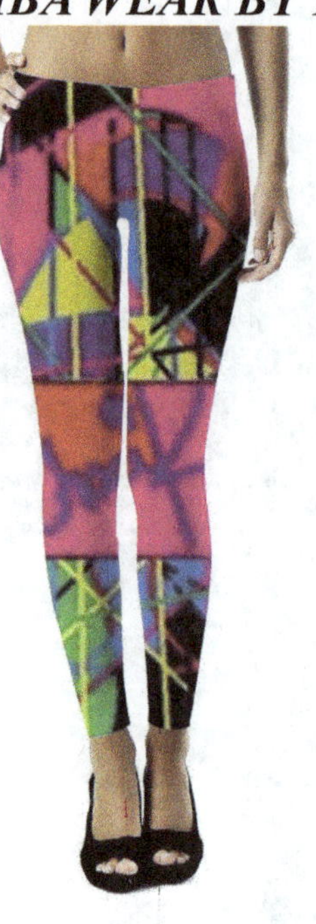

BY TRACI K COLLECTION

I am shankful for my wife and kids-Jim -VA

I am thankful for my health Liza- NC

I am thankful for surviving cancer-Traci OH

I am thankful for your smile Harold-RI

What can I say I can't complain - Ronald WI

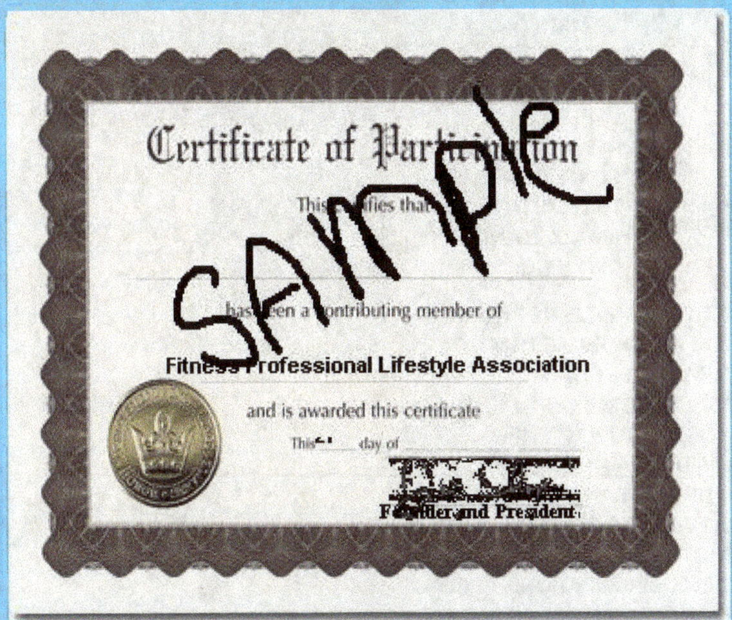

earn on of these for only $25

ARE YOU A MEMBER YET?

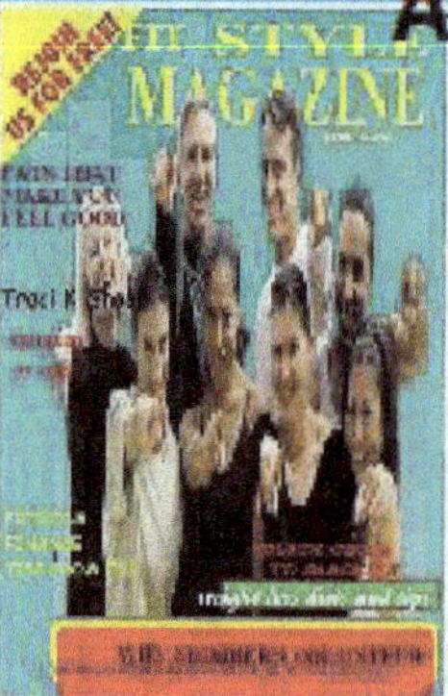

IF YOU ARE NOT A MEMBER OF FPLA FITNESS PROFESSIONAL LIFESTYLE ASSOCIATION GET GOING DON'T WAIT THE BENEFITS ARE AMAZING AND GROWING.

IF YOU THINK NOT I MEAN IT IS NOT ABOUT YOU ONLY IF YOU ARE SHOWING THAT YOU ARE ABOUT PROMOTING YOU. WEBS.COM HAS SPONSORED OUR ASSOCIATION FOR THIS TO HAPPEN YOU REGISTER AND GET A FREE MINI WEBPAGE AND UPGRADE AND GET MORE SCENE WITH A CHANCE TO GET IN ON MANY PROGRAMS. SHOWCASE YOUR BUSINESS, EXPERTISE, GET RECOMMENDATIONS, APPLY FOR ONLINE PROJECTS AND JOBS, NETWORK AND TELL OTHERS ABOUT YOURSELF, SEEN BY EDITORS, PHOTOGRAPHERS, POST YOUR NEWS ETC...

PICTURE YOURSELF FIT IN FITSTYLE MAGAZINE!

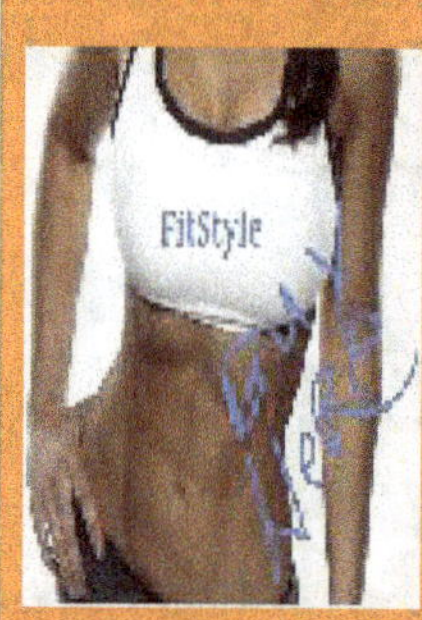

The competition is heating up more and more are entering the FITSTYLE MAGAZINE MODEL SEARCH TO BE CROWNED THIS YEARS KINGS AND QUEENS and be featured in the magazine for a chance to get tons of sponsorships opportunities

If you haven't entered yet. Show us your Fitstyle Body. How to enter go online to our cafepress and purchase your favorite FPLA item. Have a photo done and send it in or register online if you are a member put it in the photo section and then have everyone vote. They have to register to vote. www.cafepress.com/fpla

register www.fitprolifestyle.webs.com

START NOW
WWW.FITPROLIFESTYLE.WEBS.COM AND LIKE US ON FACEBOOK

JOIN OUR TEAM

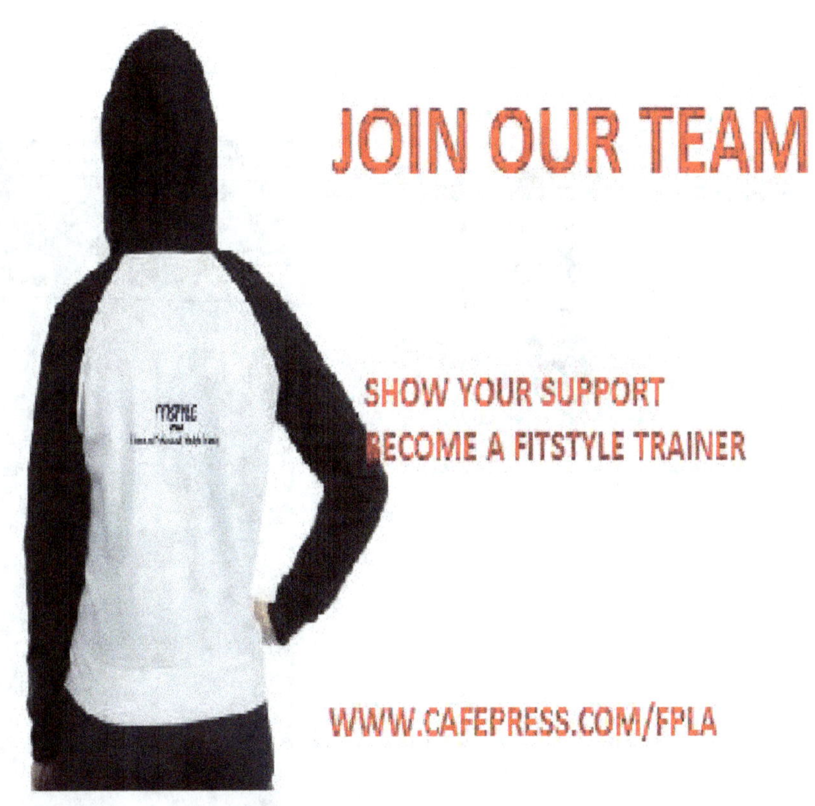

SHOW YOUR SUPPORT

BECOME A FITSTYLE TRAINER

WWW.CAFEPRESS.COM/FPLA

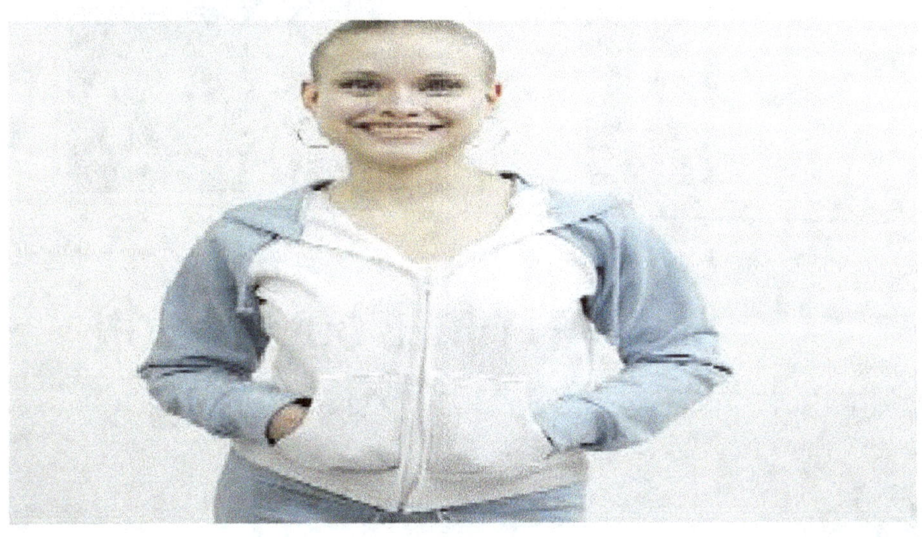

WEAR YOUR FITSTYLE CLOTHING TO SHOW SUPPORT

TAKE 20% OFF YOUR

ORDER
TODAY
CODE:
EXPLOREVIDA

FEATURED COLLECTION
TRACI K COLLECTION

WANT YOUR COLLECTION
FEATURED CONTACT US

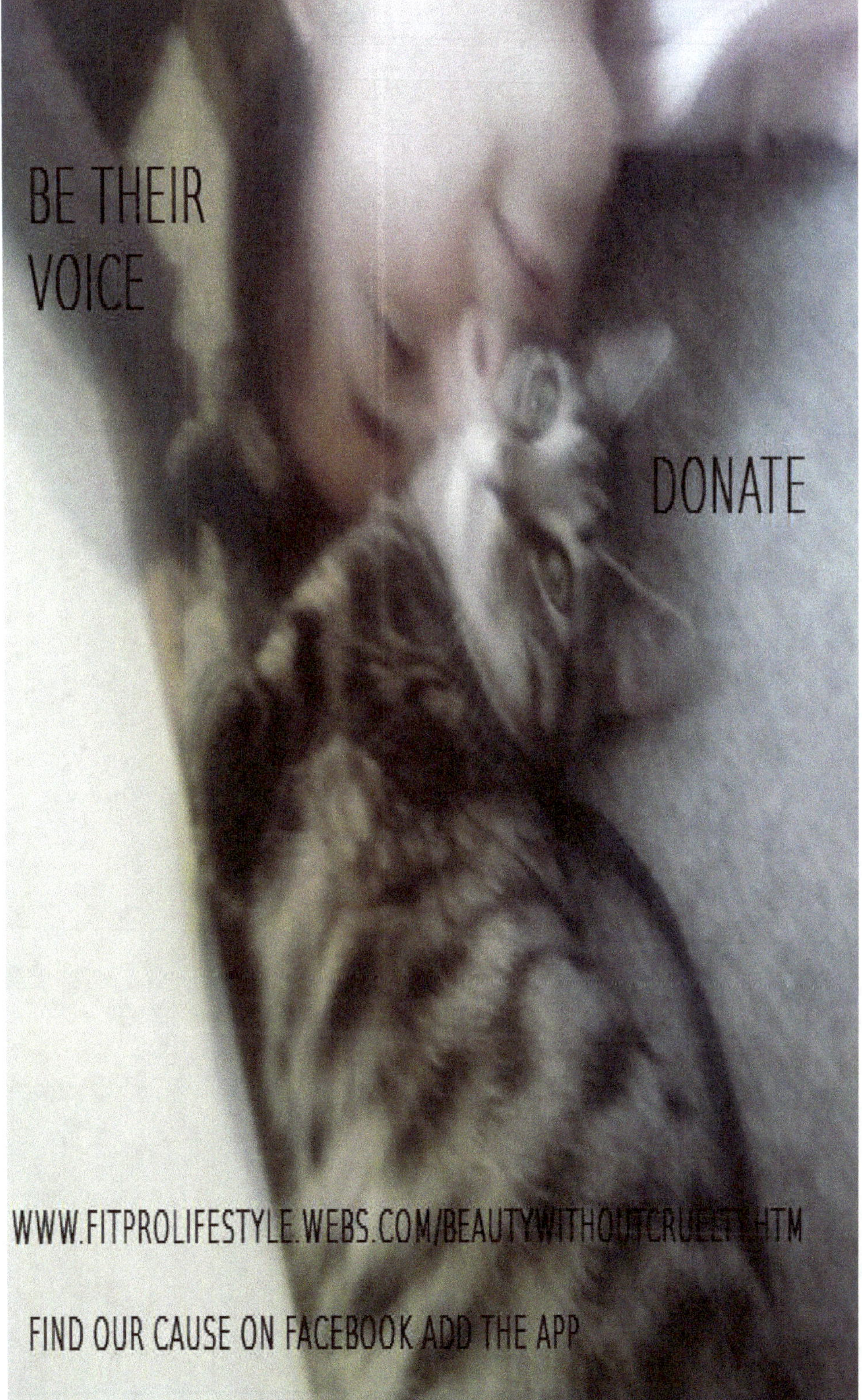
BE THEIR
VOICE
DONATE
WWW.FITPROLIFESTYLE.WEBS.COM/BEAUTYWITHOUTCRUELTY.HTM
FIND OUR CAUSE ON FACEBOOK ADD THE APP

Earn Extra Cash Online.....

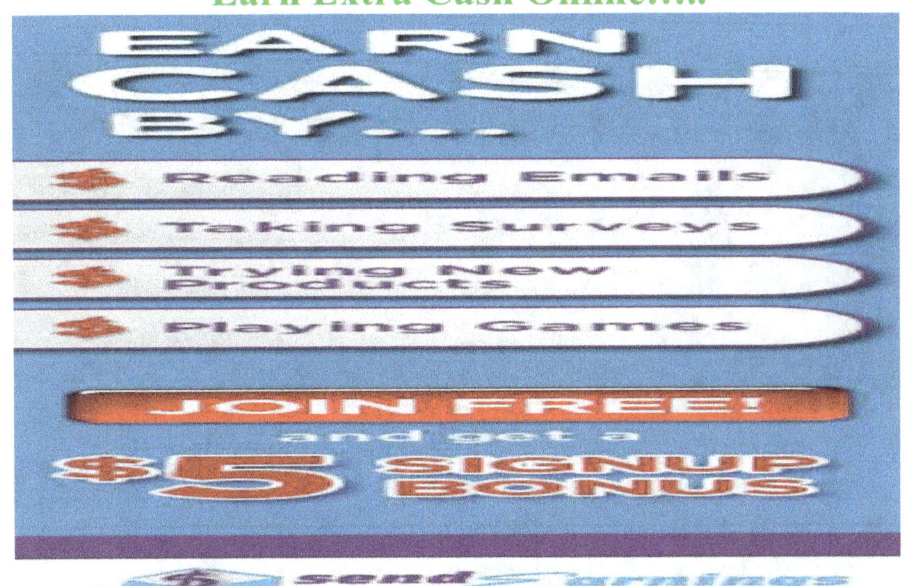

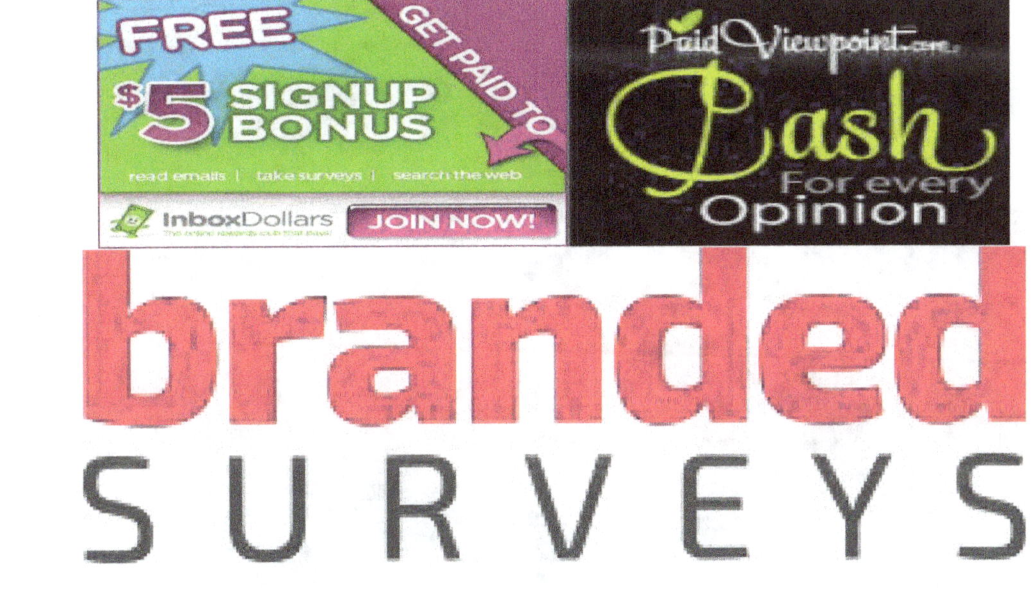

branded SURVEYS

SEE YOUR AD HERE FOR

$275 HELP WITH GET A LIFE FUND

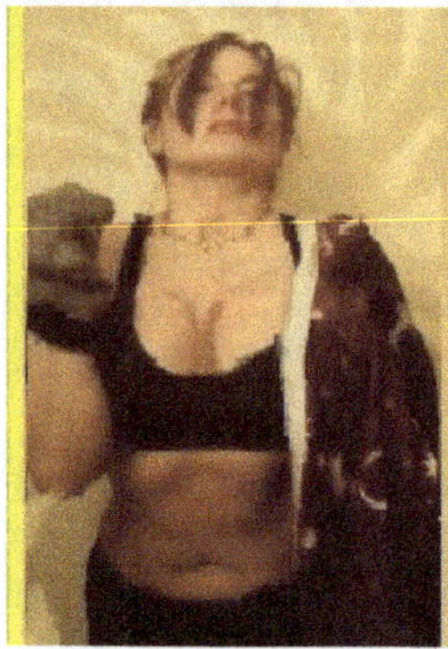

VALUE

GET CLOSER TO THAT
SIX-PACK WITH THE HELP
OF THESE LOCAL PROS.

PHOTOGRAPHED BY MICHAEL NEVEUX

1 BOX WITH LEG EXTENSION

Start in box position, with hands, knees and toes on floor and your spine in neutral.

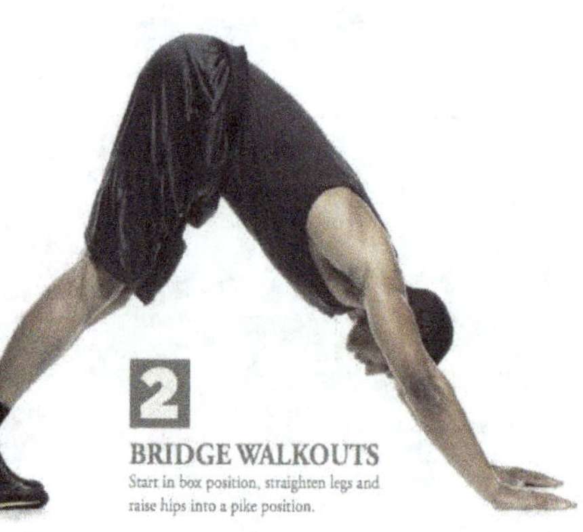

2 BRIDGE WALKOUTS

Start in box position, straighten legs and raise hips into a pike position.

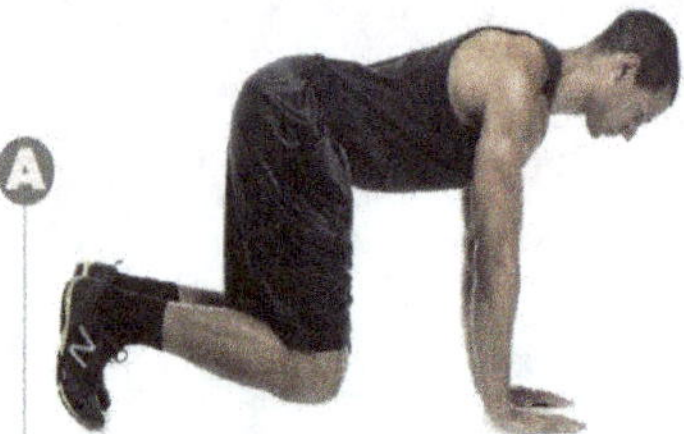

A Lift knees slightly off floor. Allow weight shift to upper back and hands. Hold for 15-30 seconds. Practice breathing calmly and chest up.

Walk hands as far away from body as possible without losing neutral spine.

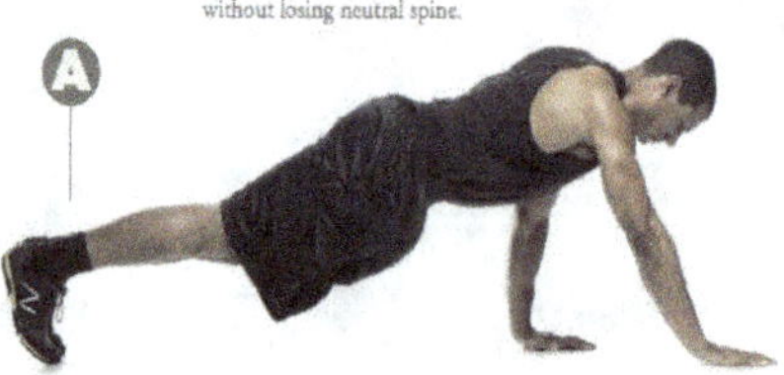

A Work to maintain calm breath and keep chest up. Hold for a beat; walk hands back to start.

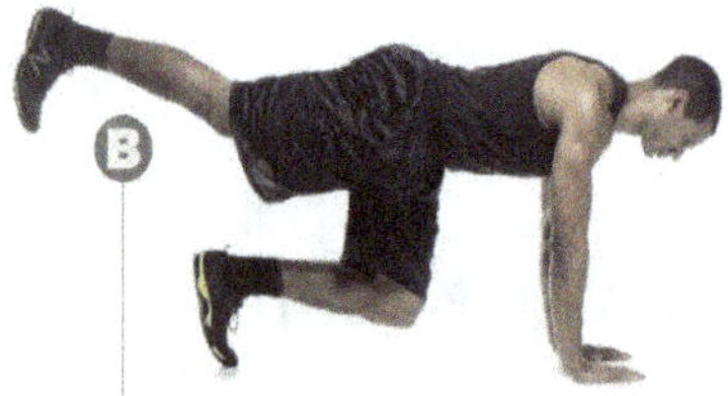

B Progress to leg extensions. Lift and push one leg back while maintaining neutral spine and breath. Alternate legs for reps.

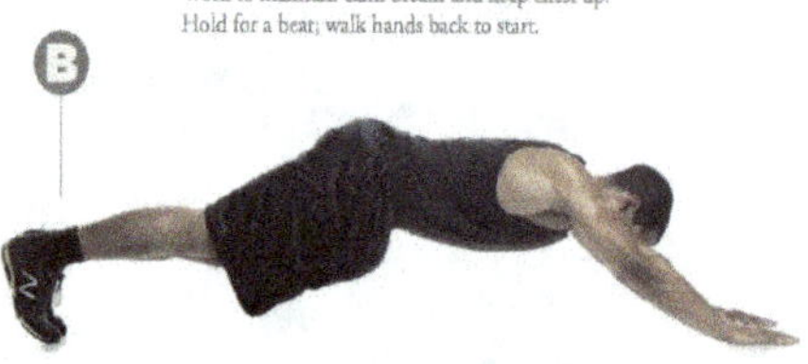

B Repeat for conditioning. You may also hold for time as a long lever plank or include push-ups between each rep.

ERIC WELDON
SPECTRUM ATHLETIC CLUB, SOUTH BAY
Strength advocate

CORE

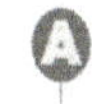

1 KNEE UP TWIST

Set up in a full plank position with your hands underneath your shoulders and legs long. Pull your right knee to your nose (make sure to pull your abdominals up and away from your thigh).

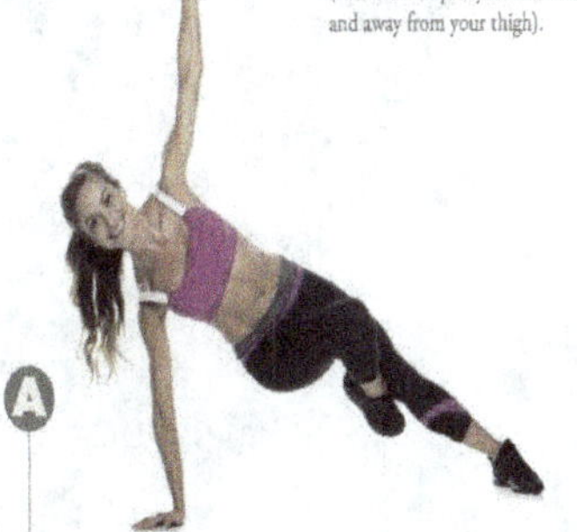

A

Transition to a side plank, putting all the weight into your right arm, turning to the inside of the left foot and reaching left arm to sky. Continue to pull right knee to nose.

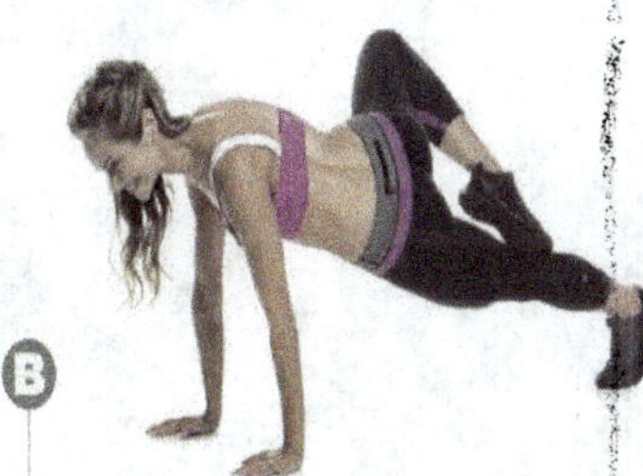

B

Lower the left hand and return to plank with knee drawn in, then externally rotate leg to open knee out to right. Try to get right leg parallel with floor. Hold for a moment and return to start, step back to plank and repeat with opposite leg.

Alternate legs for 10-15 reps total.

2 STACKED V-UP

Lie on the floor with hands behind your head and elbows wide. Stack your left leg on top of your right leg. Press your heel of left foot and toes of right foot into each other to engage inner thighs.

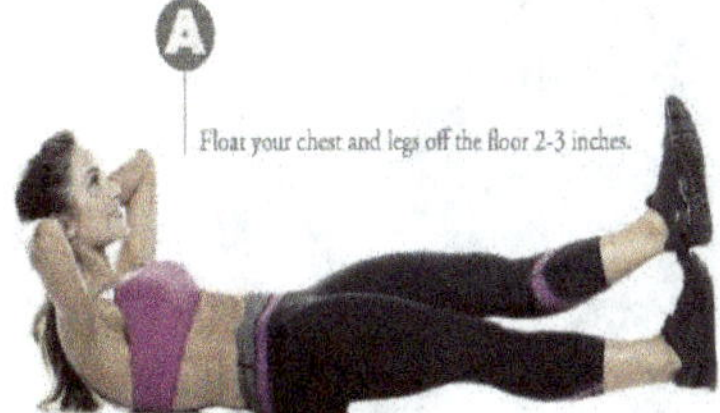

A

Float your chest and legs off the floor 2-3 inches.

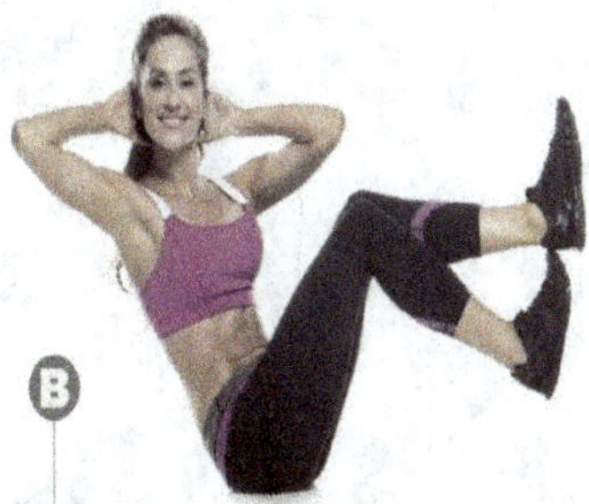

B

Begin to pull your knees into your chest, while sitting up and lifting the entire back off floor. At the same time twist away from the top leg, reaching left elbow outside right knee. Return to movement A, never returning all the way to the ground until you complete 10-15 reps each side.

CHRISTINE BULLOCK
EQUINOX, MANHATTAN BEACH
Pilates, yoga, group fitness instructor, prenatal and postnatal exercise consultant, health and wellness nutrition consultant
christinebullock.com

FIT STYLE MAGAZINE

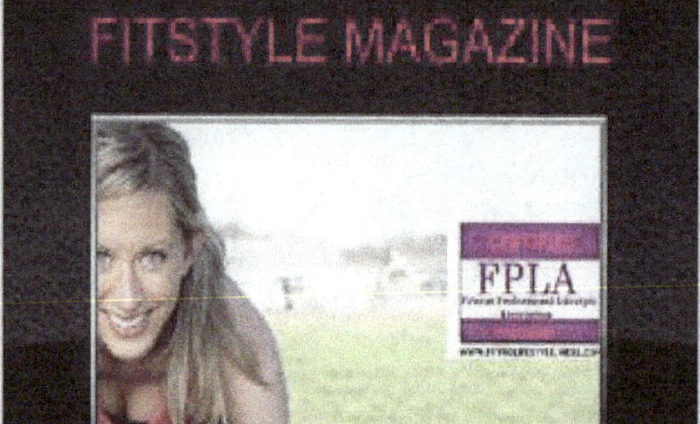

COVER CALENDAR

GET IT NOW!

CONGRATULATIONS

SUPPORT FITSTYLE $25

ON SALE

*WORKING IT OUT *
THE MOVIE

LIKE

WWW.FACEBOOK.COM/WORKINGITOUTTHEMOVIE

MOST BEAUTIFUL PEOPLE OF HEALTH

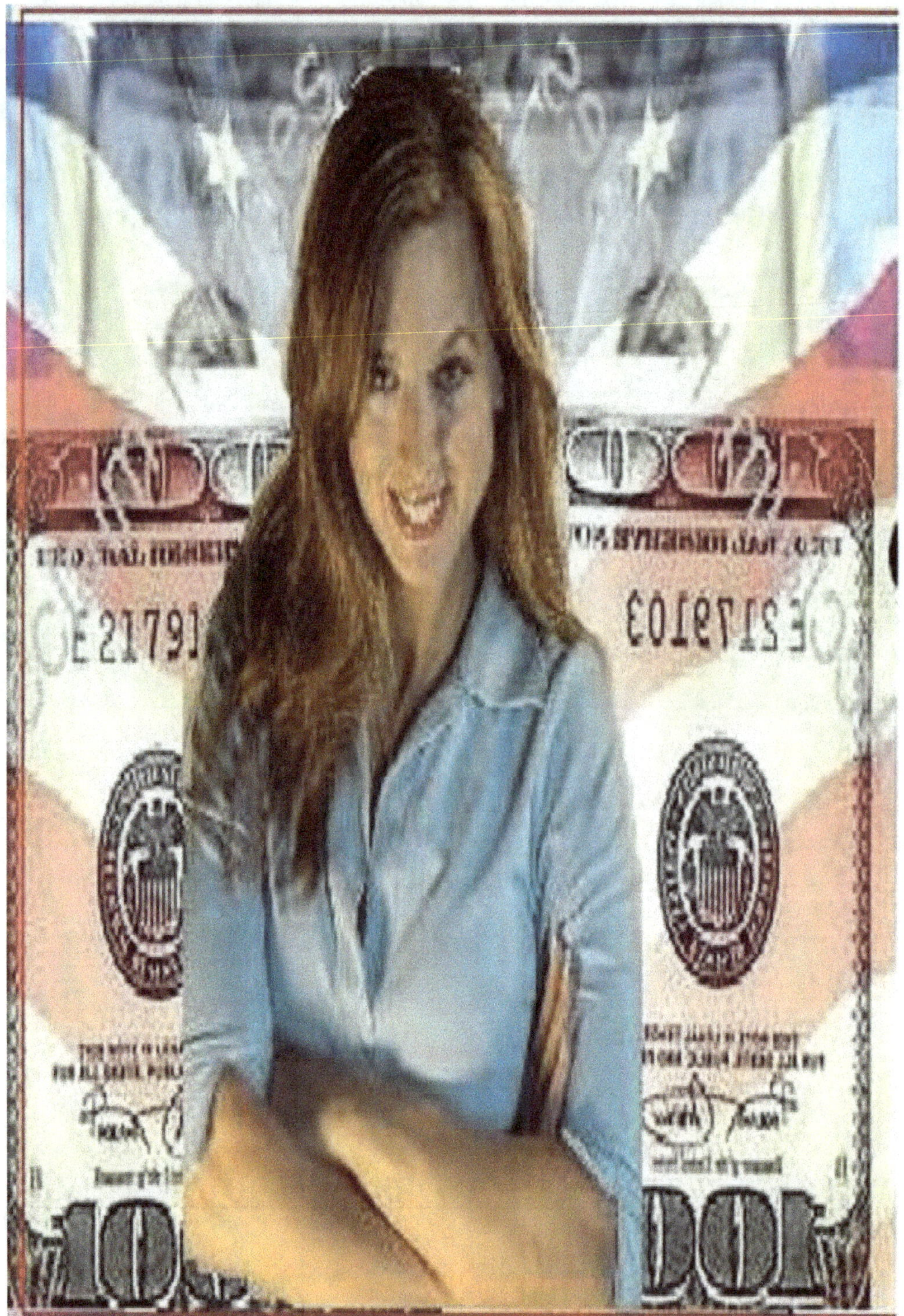

VOTE NOW AND RANK

FITSTYLE YOUR BEST REALITY
AT HOME....SOON

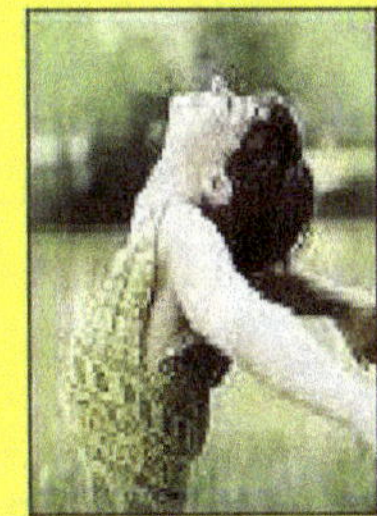

WORKOUTS

SHOOTOUTS

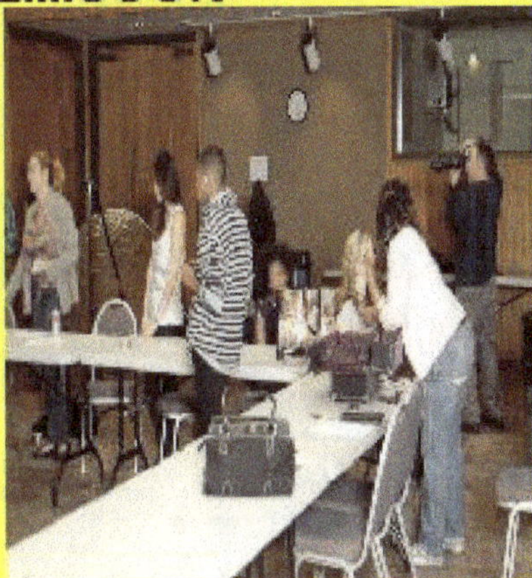

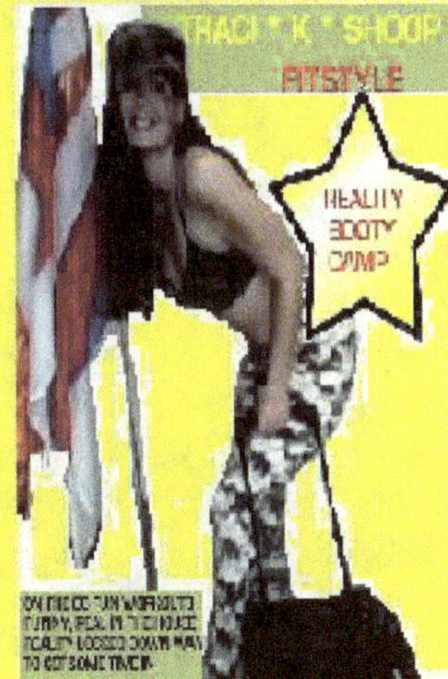

BOOTY CAMP dvd SETS

SUBSCRIBE TO BE FEATURED MEMBER

www.youtube.com/fitstylemag

GET FREE EBOOKS

WHEN YOU BECOME A MEMBER

TO USE IN YOUR CAREER OR LIFESTYLE

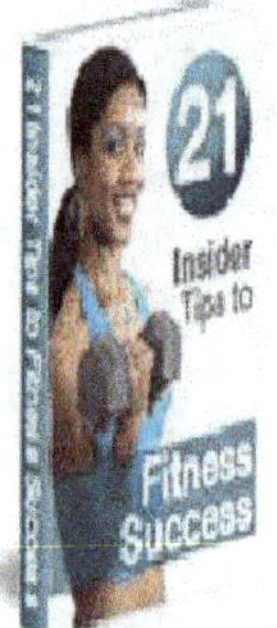

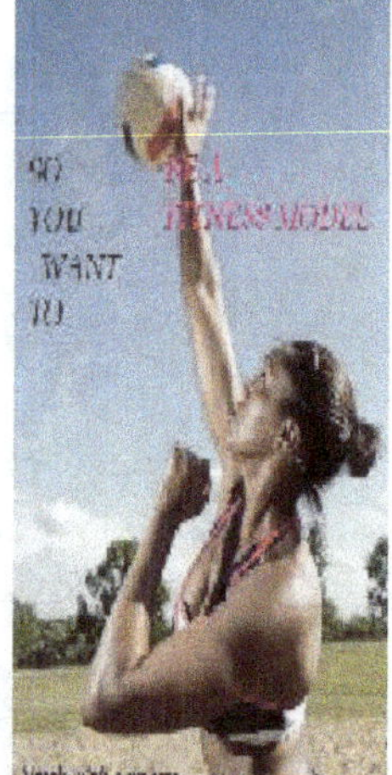

FAT CHANCE

SO YOU WANT TO
BE A FITNESS
MODEL
DONATION $

TRUTH ABOUT WEIGHT LOSS SUPPLEMENTS

BONUS

5 MUST KNOW AB EXERCISES

TO GIVE TO YOUR CLIENTS

REGISTER NOW!

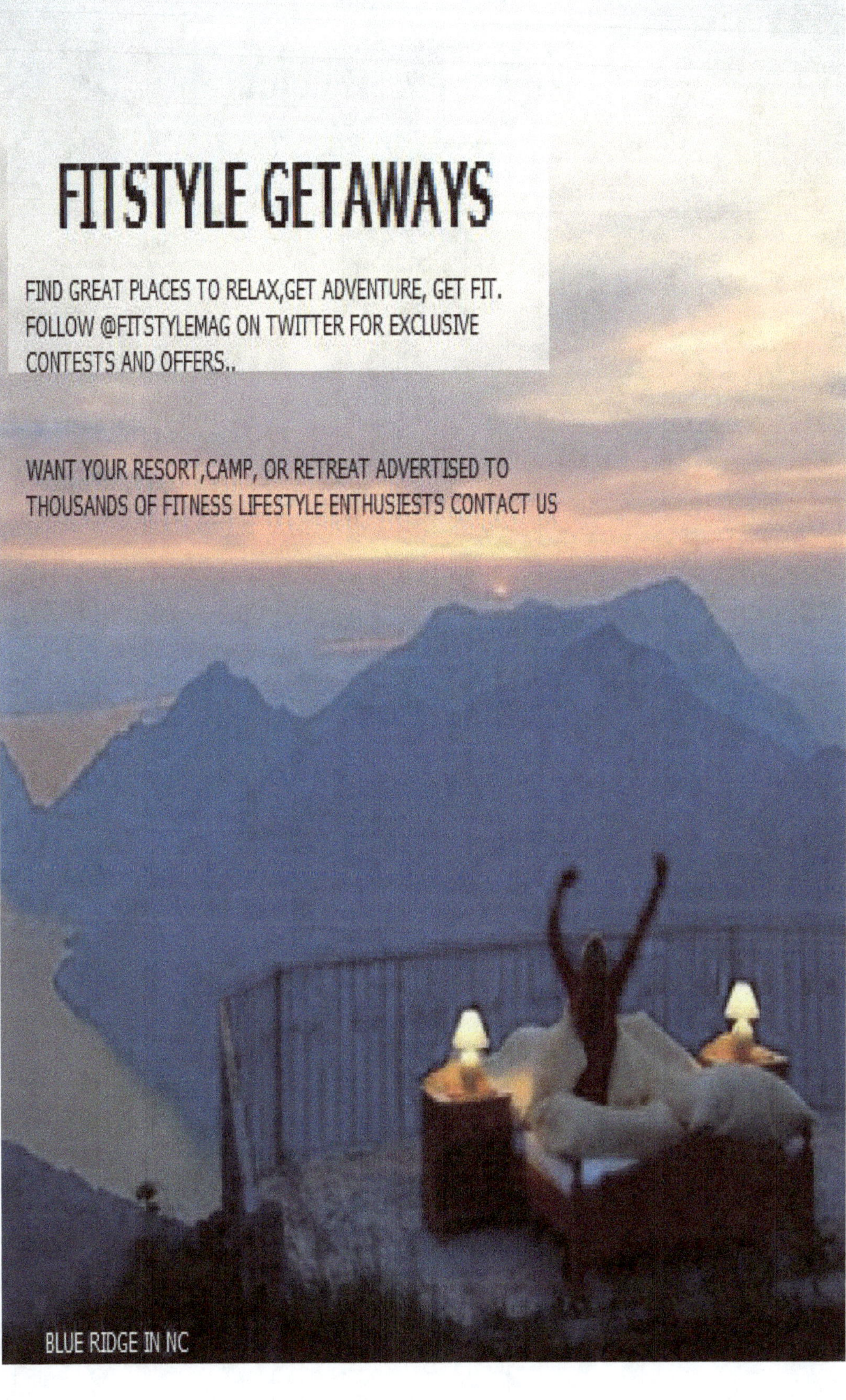

FITSTYLE GETAWAYS
FIND GREAT PLACES TO RELAX,GET ADVENTURE, GET FIT.
FOLLOW @FITSTYLEMAG ON TWITTER FOR EXCLUSIVE
CONTESTS AND OFFERS..
WANT YOUR RESORT,CAMP, OR RETREAT ADVERTISED TO
THOUSANDS OF FITNESS LIFESTYLE ENTHUSIESTS CONTACT US
BLUE RIDGE IN NC

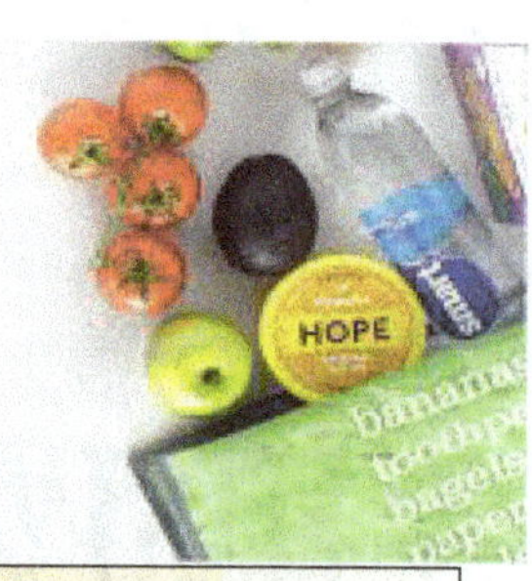

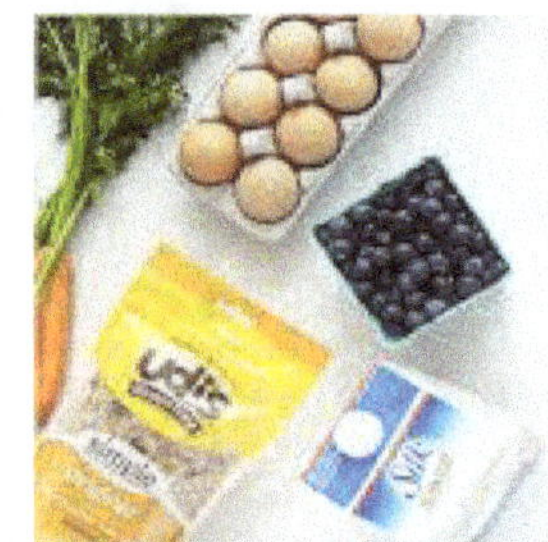

MAGAZINE
GOT A BLOG GET A FEATURE FOR $25
WWW.GIRLIEGIRLLOVE.BLOGSPOT.COM

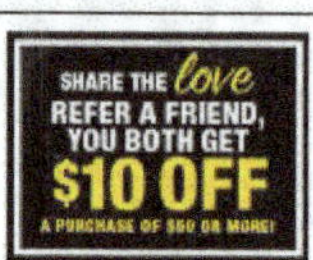

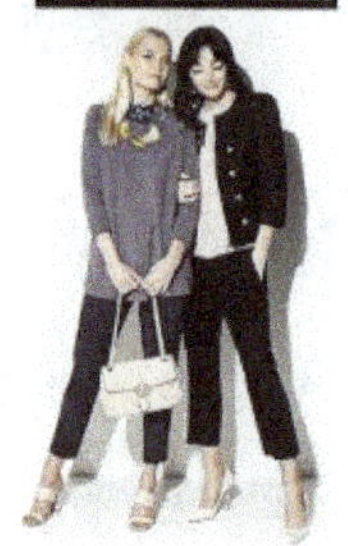

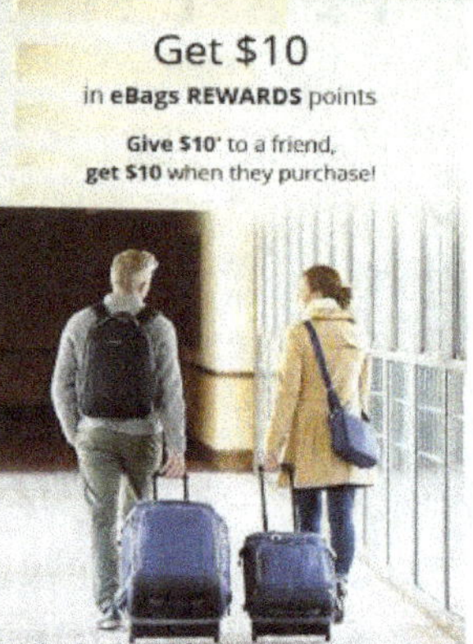

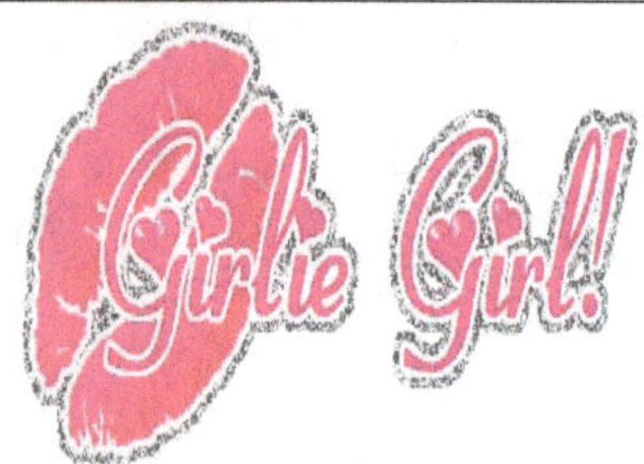

Get $5 simple and FREE

$15 TO SHOP
REFER A FRIEND
GET ANOTHER $15

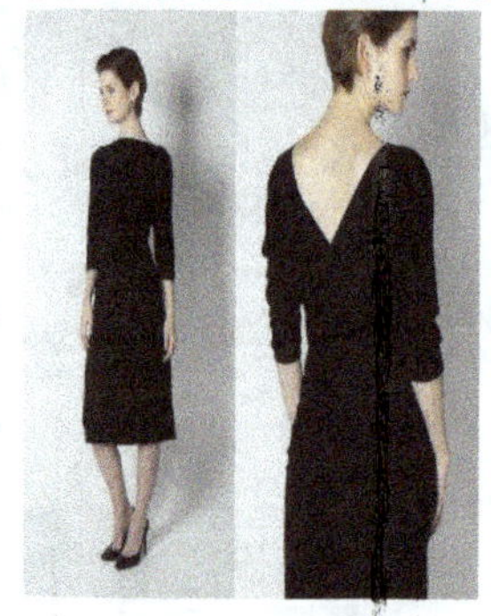

EARN POINTS
REFER GET MORE
AND THEN
PAYOUT

YOUR

AD

**HERE
CONTACT US**

JGFCGROUP@AOL.COM

YOUR

AD

**HERE
CONTACT US**

JGFCGROUP@AOL.COM

YOUR

AD

**HERE
CONTACT US**

JGFCGROUP@AOL.COM

FITSTYLE FINE JEWELRY

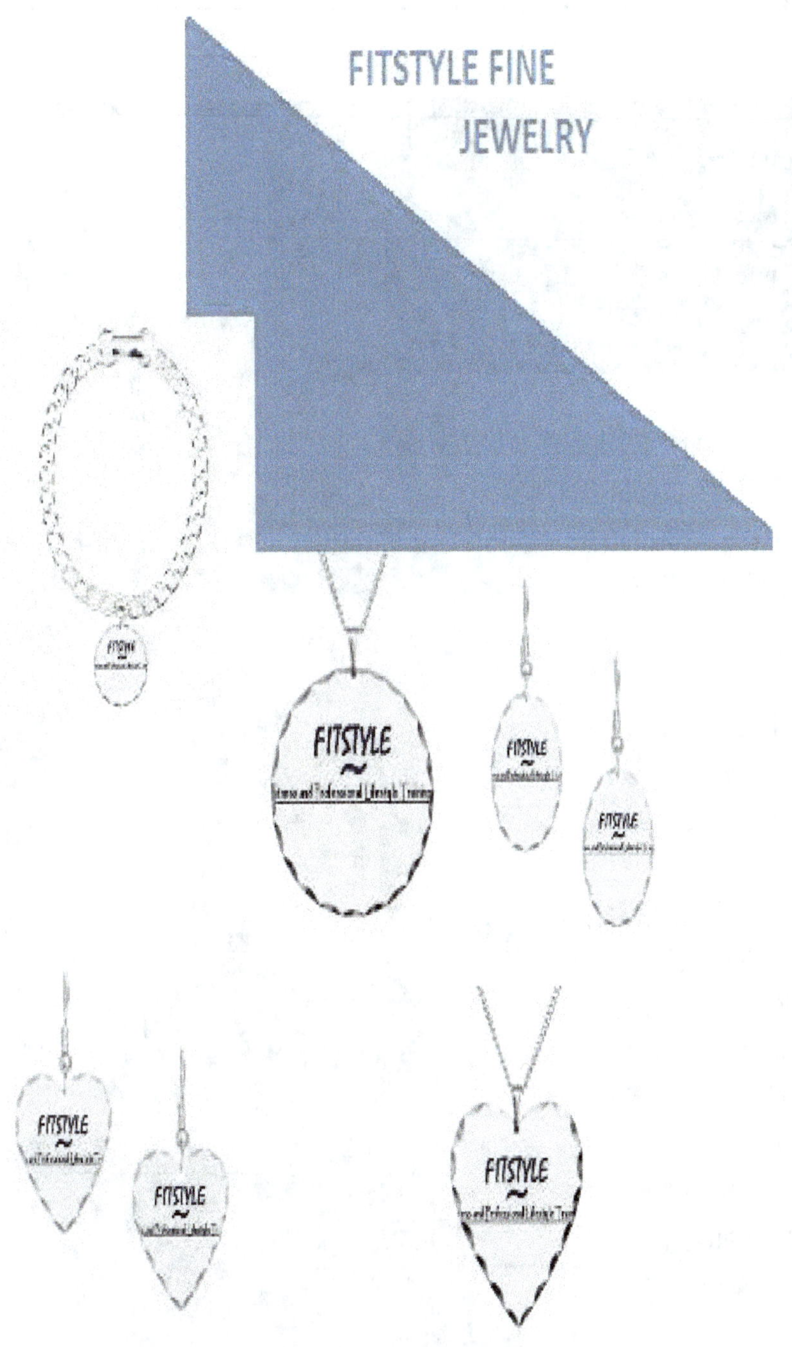

RANGE FROM $16.99-$30.00

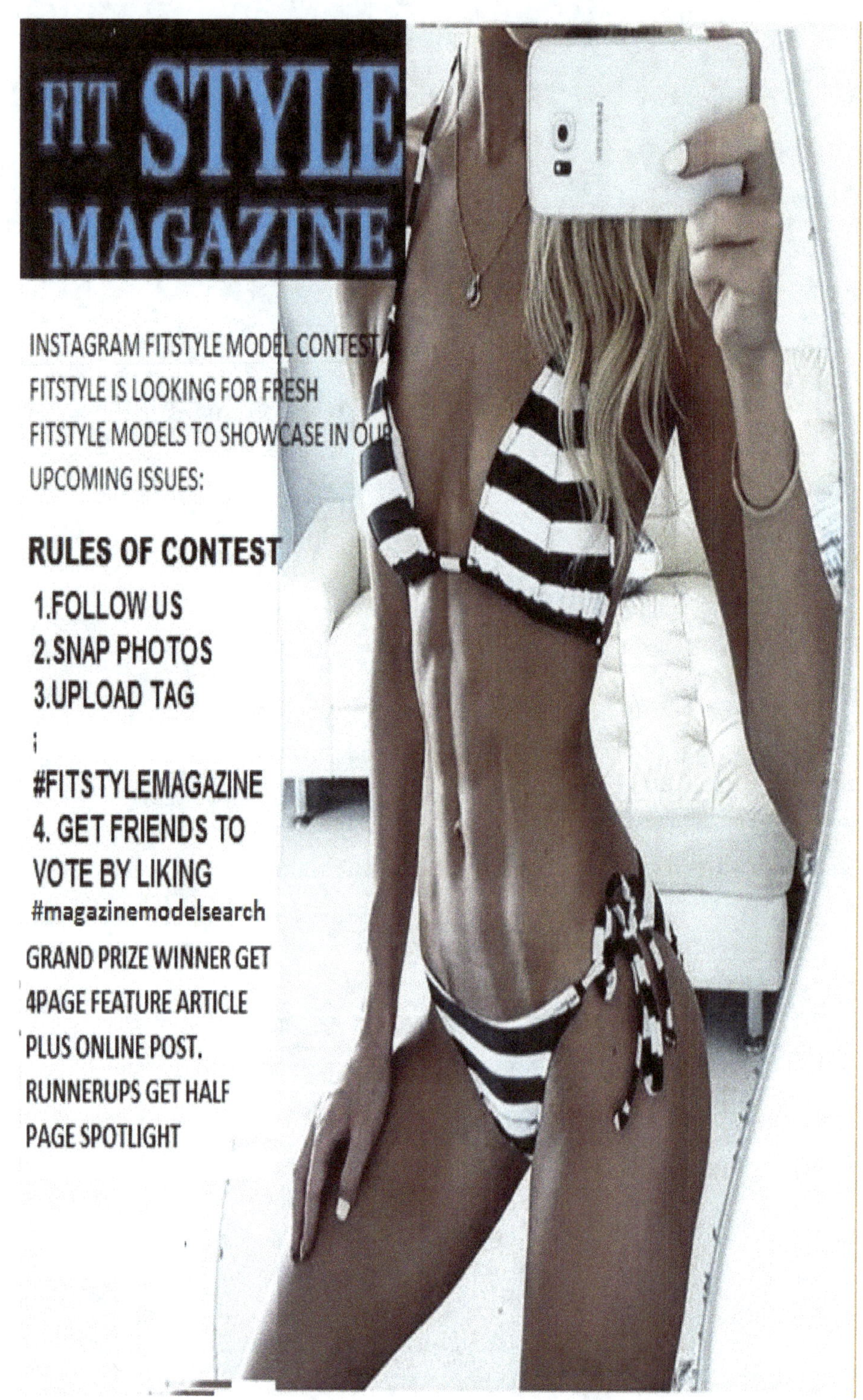
FIT STYLE MAGAZINE

INSTAGRAM FITSTYLE MODEL CONTEST
FITSTYLE IS LOOKING FOR FRESH
FITSTYLE MODELS TO SHOWCASE IN OUR
UPCOMING ISSUES:

RULES OF CONTEST
1.FOLLOW US
2.SNAP PHOTOS
3.UPLOAD TAG

#FITSTYLEMAGAZINE
4. GET FRIENDS TO
VOTE BY LIKING
#magazinemodelsearch
GRAND PRIZE WINNER GET
4PAGE FEATURE ARTICLE
PLUS ONLINE POST.
RUNNERUPS GET HALF
PAGE SPOTLIGHT

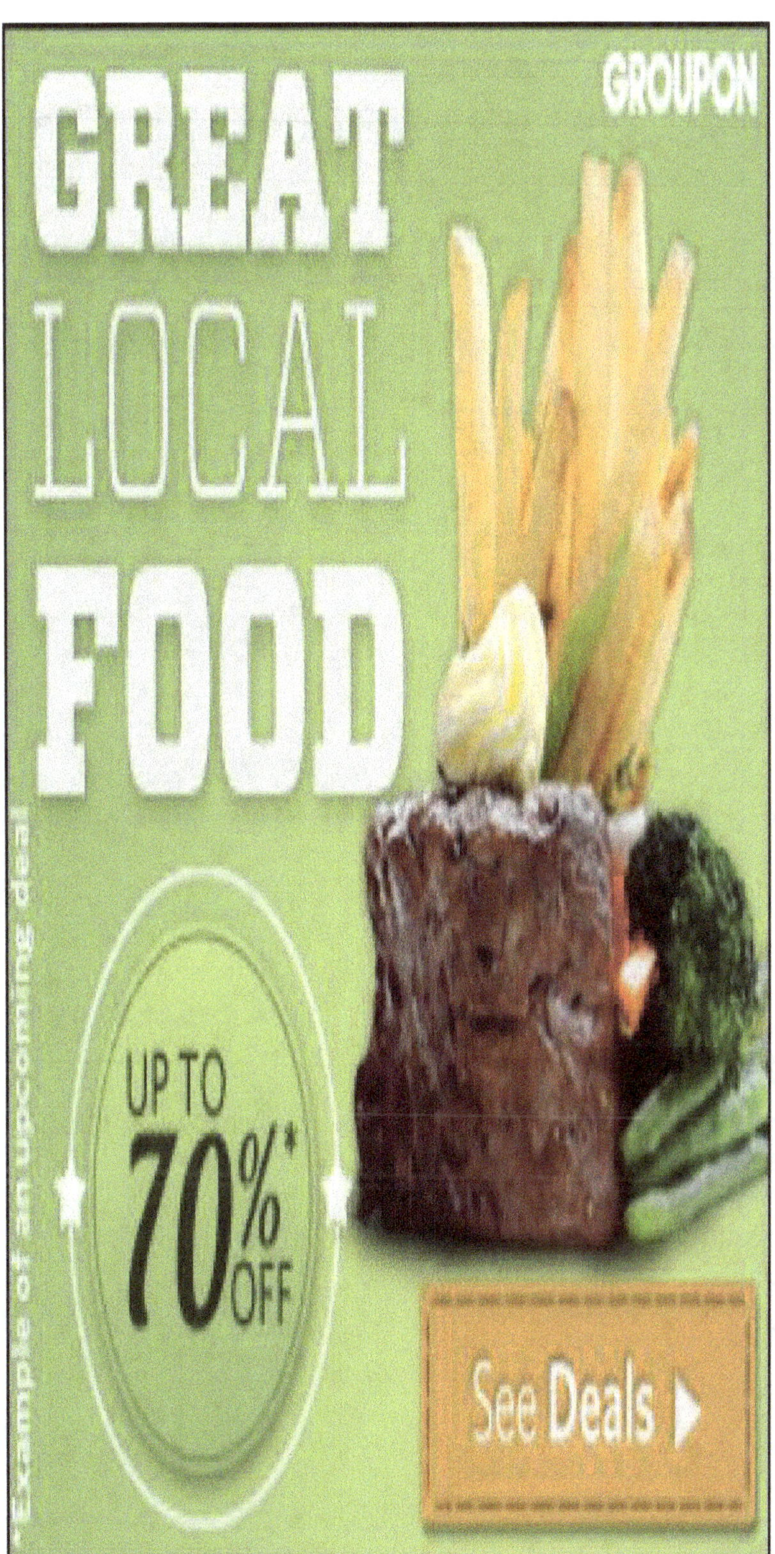

GROUPON
GREAT
LOCAL
FOOD
UP TO
70%*
OFF
See Deals
*Example of an upcoming deal

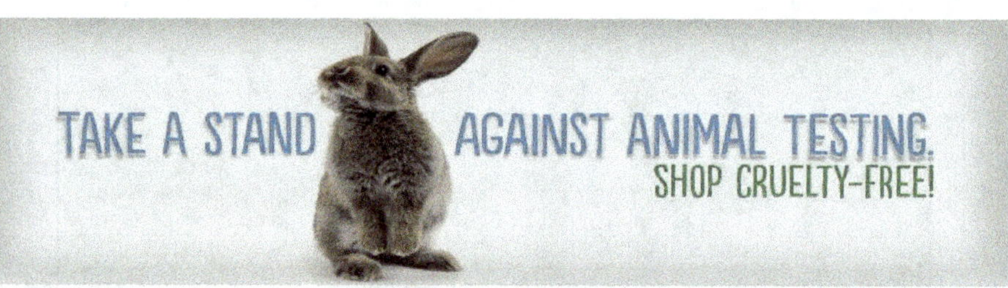

Where to Buy Cruelty Free Makeup

Sephora

Anastasia Beverly Hills
Ardency Inn
bareMinerals ^
beautyblender
BECCA
Besame Cosmetics
Bite Beauty
butter LONDON
Cinema Secrets
Cover FX *
Deborah Lippman
DERMAdoctor
Embryolisse
Eyeko
Hourglass
jINsoon
Josie Maran
Kat Von D
Koh Gen Do
LAVANILA *
Lit Cosmetics
Living Proof
Nails Inc
NARS ^
NUDE skincare
NUDESTIX
Obsessive Compulsive Cosmetics *
Perfekt Beauty
Sunday Riley
Supergoop!
tarte ^
TokyoMilk Dark
Too Faced *
Urban Decay * ~ ^
Wen *

* offers vegan products
^ parent company is not cruelty free
~ Leaping Bunny Certified

Ulta

Anastasia Beverly Hills
bareMinerals ^
Burt's Bees ^ ~
BECCA
butter LONDON
CeraVe
Deborah Lippman
DermOrganic *
ecoTools *
Freeman ^
It Cosmetics
Juice Beauty
Mineral Fusion *
Marc Anthony
Mally Beauty
Nails Inc
Nyx ^
Orly
Pacifica *
Paul Mitchell ~
Pureology *
Pur Minerals
Reviva Labs
Real Techniques
Tarte ^
The Body Shop ^ ~
Too Faced *
Urban Decay * ~ ^
Yes to

Drugstore

essence
Flower
Milani Cosmetics
Nyx Cosmetics ^
Physicians Formula
Pixi Beauty
Prestige Beauty
Wet n' Wild

Online

Cover FX *
Urban Decay * ~ ^
Makeup Geek *
Ofra Cosmetics * ~
Too Faced *
Sugarpill *
Obsessive Compulsive Cosmetics *
Fyrinnae *
Darling Girl *
Anastasia Beverly Hills
Aromaleigh
Ben Nye
Cate McNabb ~
Charlotte Tilbury
Colour Pop
Concrete Minerals *
Cult Nails *
Dose of Colors *
Dreamworld Hermetica *
e.l.f. Cosmetics
Face Atelier * ~
Femme Fatale
Glamour Doll Eyes *
Geek Chic *
glo Minerals
Hello Waffle
Illamasqua
Inglot
It Cosmetics
Jane Iredale ~
Jeffree Star *
Jesse's Girl
Josie Maran *
Life's Entropy *
Literary Lacquers
Mehron Cosmetics
Meow Cosmetics *
Melt Cosmetics *
Milani Cosmetics ~
Mineral Fusion ~ *
Morgana Cryptoria *
NARS ^
Nyx Cosmetics ^
Performance Colors
Perfekt Beauty
Purely Cosmetics
Rituel de Fille
Rouge Bunny Rouge
Saucebox Cosmetics
Senna Cosmetics
Silk Naturals *
Tarina Tarantino
Tarte ^
The All Natural Face *
Virus Insanity

Traci K Beauty

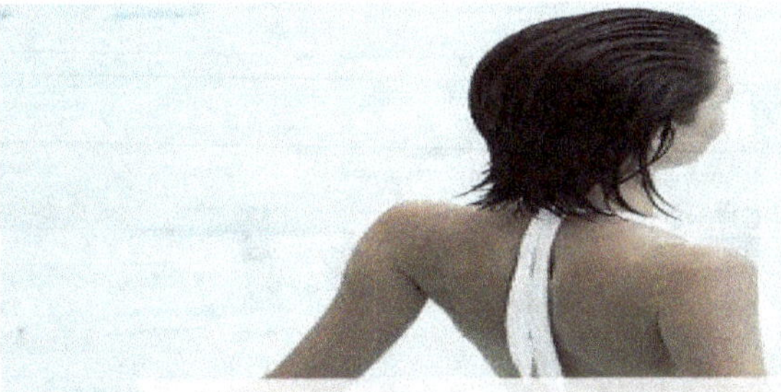

scissor skier

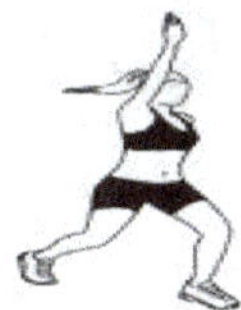 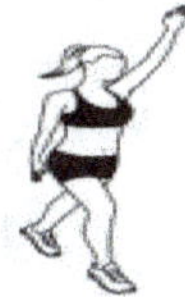

3sets 60sec

bent over lateral raise

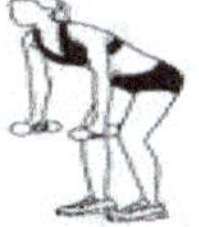 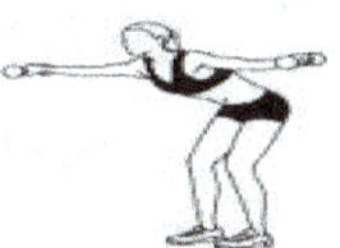

3sets 60sec

bow and arrow squat pull

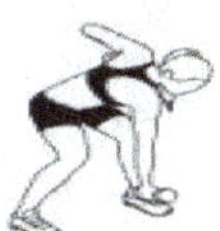 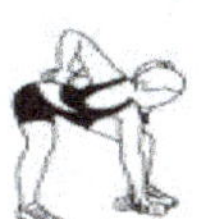

3sets 45sec

hindu push ups

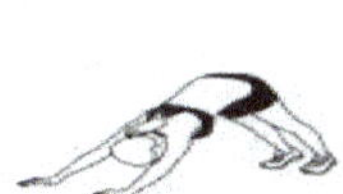 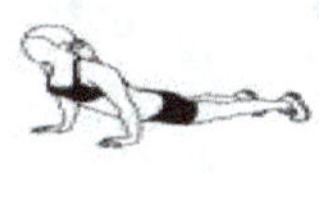

3sets 45sec

half squat jab cross

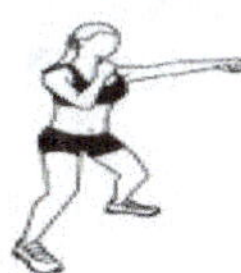 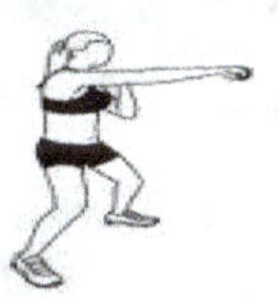

3sets 45sec

dumbbell bent over row

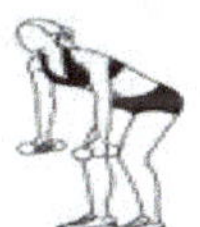 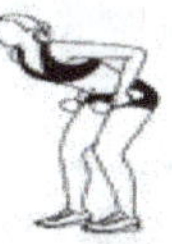

3sets 60sec

deadlift wide row

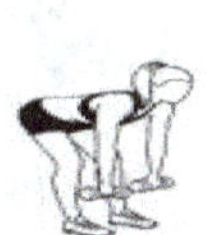 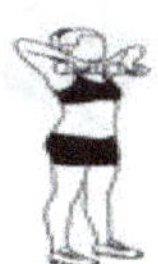

3sets 60sec

pike push up

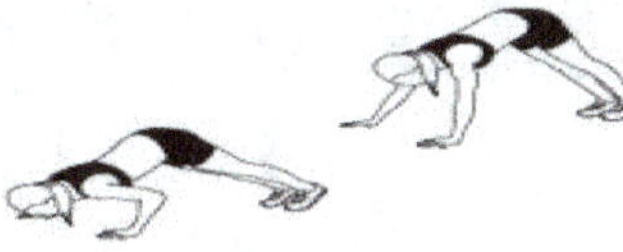

3sets 45sec

basketball shots

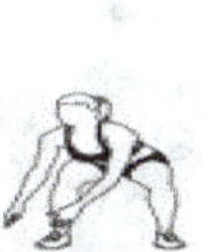 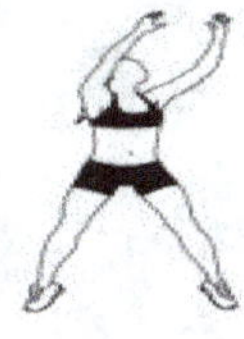

3sets 30sec + 30sec

wide row

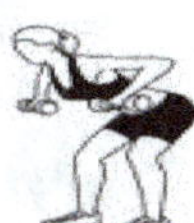 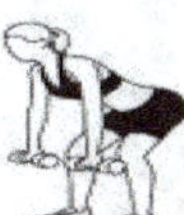

3sets 60sec

Back Workout

FitnessFoodDiva.Com

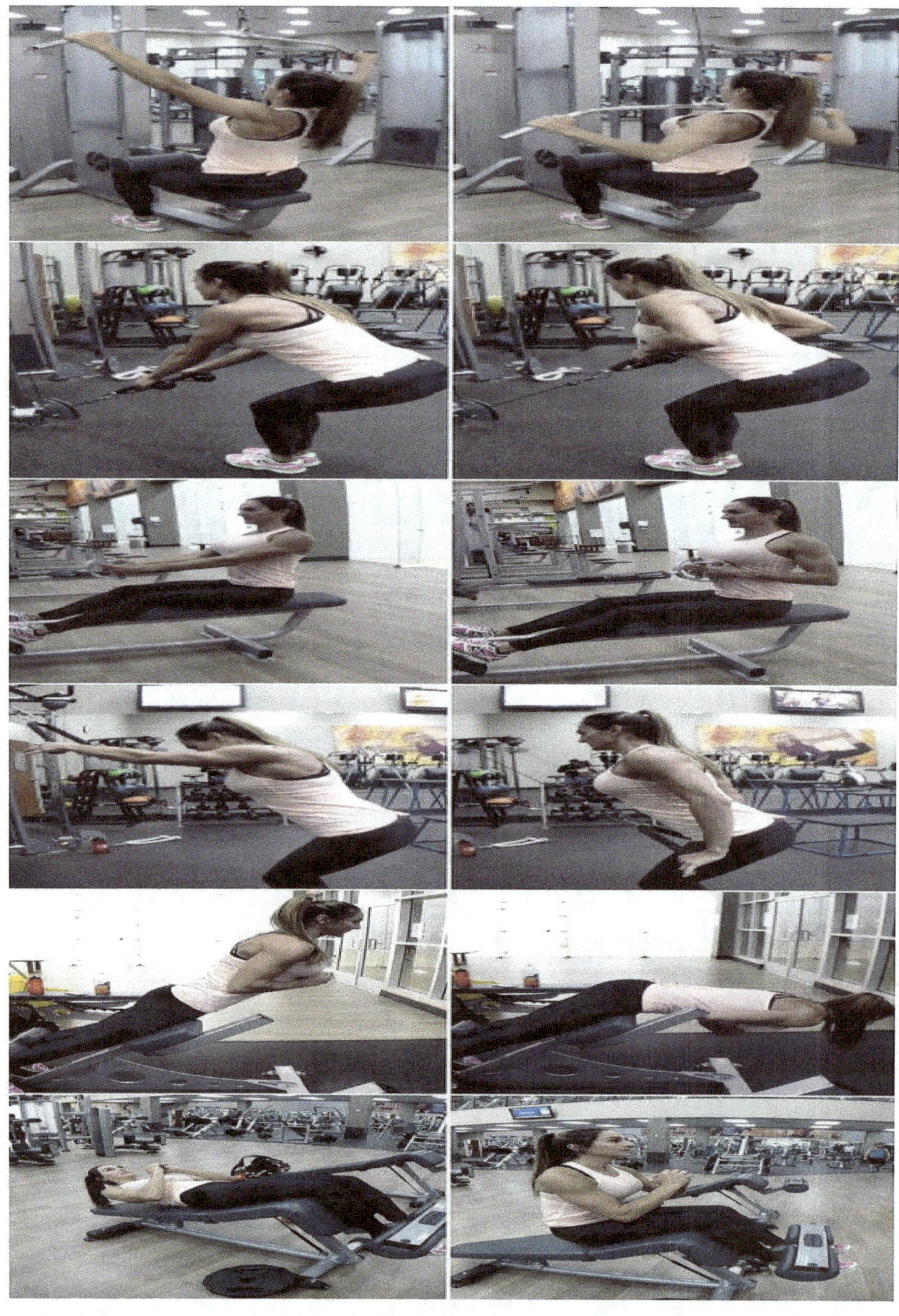

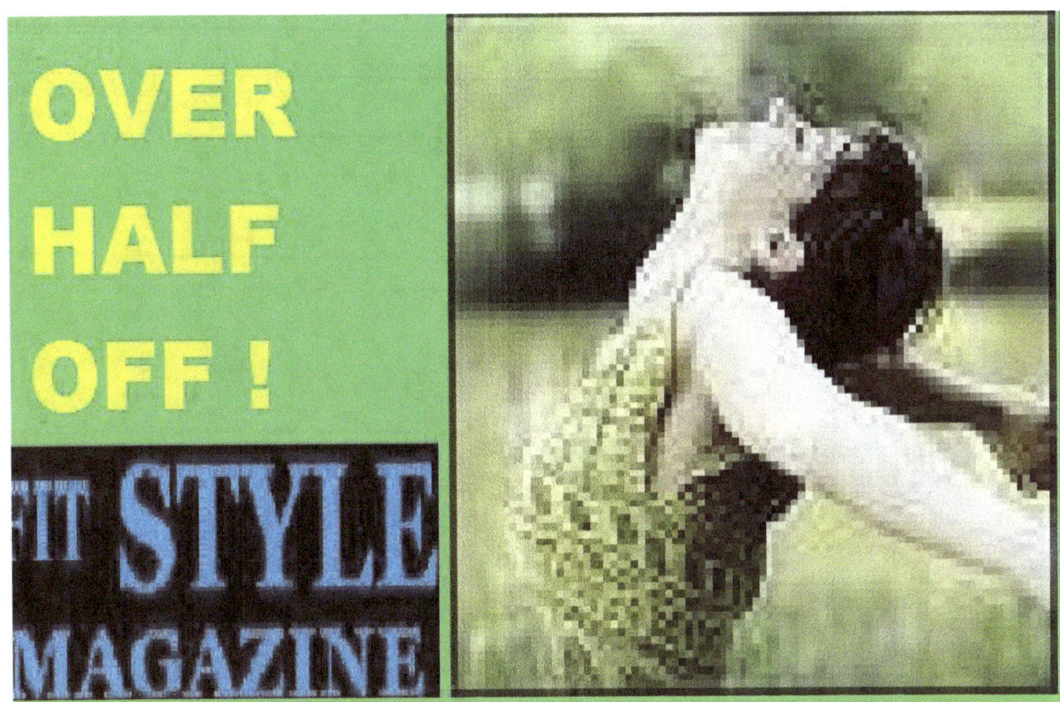

FitStyle Magazine and network provides you with tools to help you grow your client or fan base....and much more

each month you will find more resources, tips from other members, expert advice and inspiration articles to help you achieve goals www.fitprolifestyle.webs.com

COMING THIS SUMMER IN OHIO AND CITIES LIKE US ON FACEBOOK
TO FIND WHERE AUDITIONS WILL BE
SEE WHO WILL BE 2017 NOMINEES

HAVE AN EVENT?   LET US KNOW SPONSORS WELCOMED

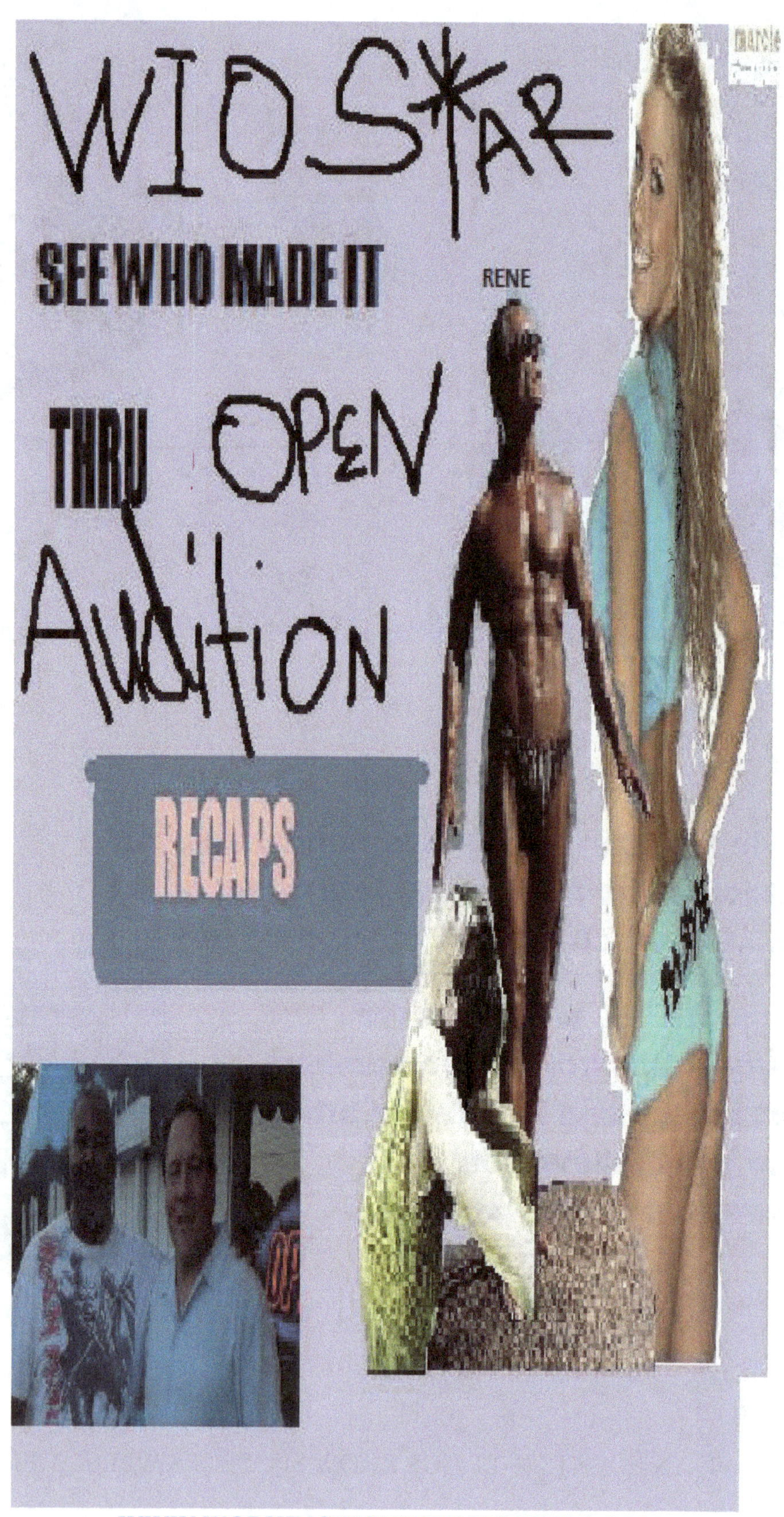
WIO STAR
SEE WHO MADE IT
RENE
THRU OPEN Audition
RECAPS

WWW.WORKINGITOUTSERIES.WEBS.COM

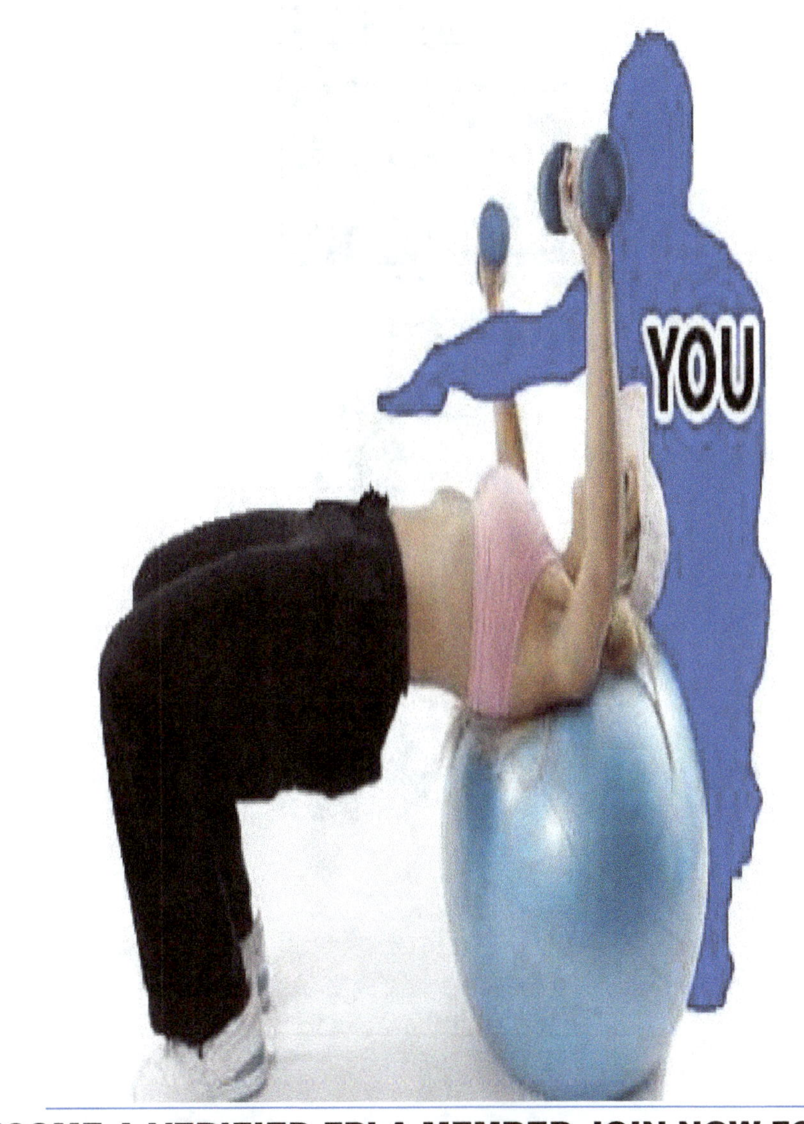

BECOME A VERIFIED FPLA MEMBER JOIN NOW FOR $25

$100 FOR DIRECTORY LISTING

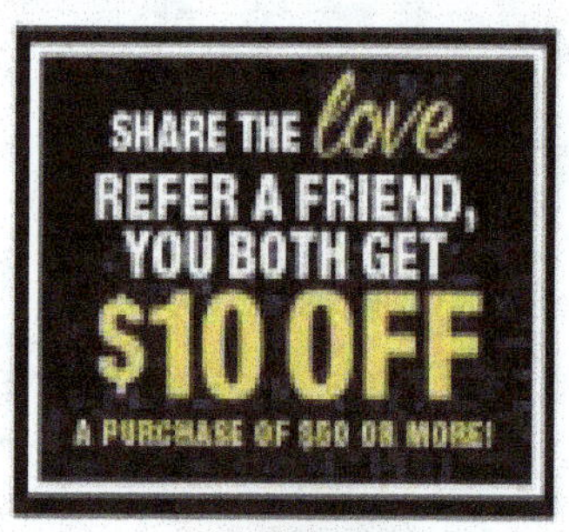

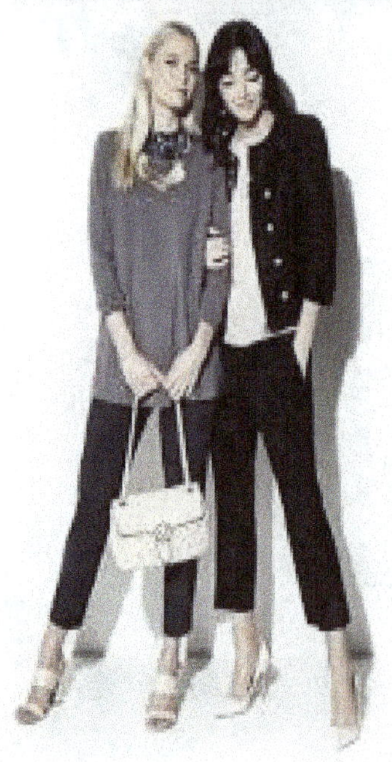

Like handbags refer to get them
https://refer.lastcall.com/s/gfcconnection

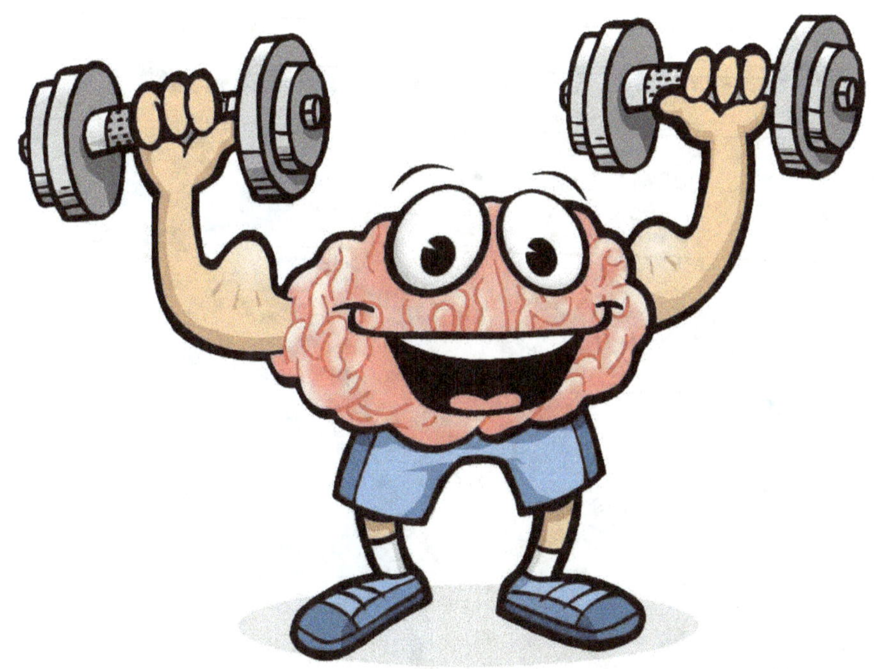

TRAIN YOUR BRAIN WITH THESE EXERCISES RECAPS FOR MAY MENTAL HEALTH AWARENESS MONTH

LEFT BRAIN FUNCTIONS

Right side of body control

Number skills

Math/Scientific skills

Analytical

Objectivity

Written language

Spoken language

Logic

Reasoning

RIGHT BRAIN FUNCTIONS

Left side of body control

3-D shapes

Music/Art awareness

Synthesizing

Subjectivity

Imagination

Intuition

Creativity

Emotion

Face recognition

THE BRAIN BENEFITS OF EXERCISE

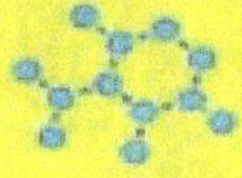 INCREASES PRODUCTION OF NEUROCHEMICALS THAT PROMOTE BRAIN CELL REPAIR

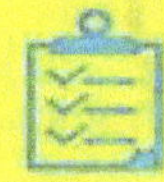 IMPROVES MEMORY

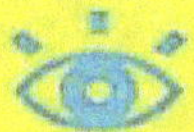 LENGTHENS ATTENTION SPAN

 BOOSTS DECISION-MAKING SKILLS

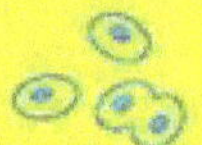 PROMPTS GROWTH OF NEW NERVE CELLS AND BLOOD VESSELS

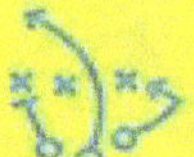 IMPROVES MULTI-TASKING AND PLANNING

7 Ways to Keep Your Brain Healthy as You Age

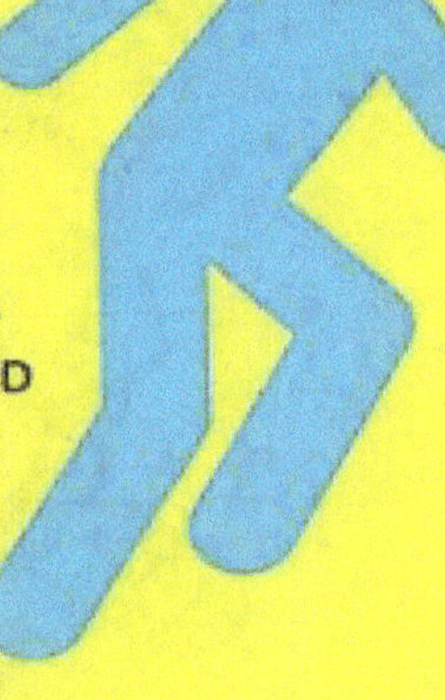

1. Build up cognitive reserve by learning something new or a new language.

2. Monitor your blood sugar. Diabetes is linked w/ a higher risk of dementia.

3. Keep your blood pressure within the recommended range. High blood pressure damages blood vessels in the brain.

4. Aerobic exercise helps your brain form new connections. Get your heart rate up for 20 min. + a few times per week.

5. Protect your head against injury. Head injuries increase the risk of dementia.

6. Take sugar & refined carbs out of your diet. They're linked w/ inflammation. Add more plant-based foods to your plate.

7. Make sure you're getting enough B-vitamins in your diet. Vitamin B12 is especially important for cognitive health.

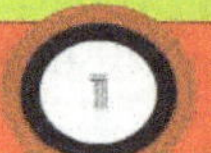
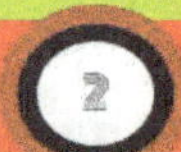
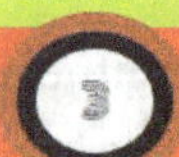
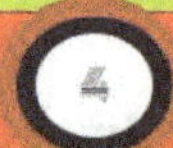
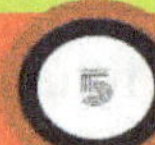
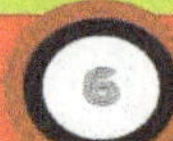
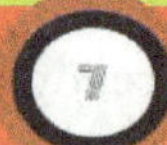
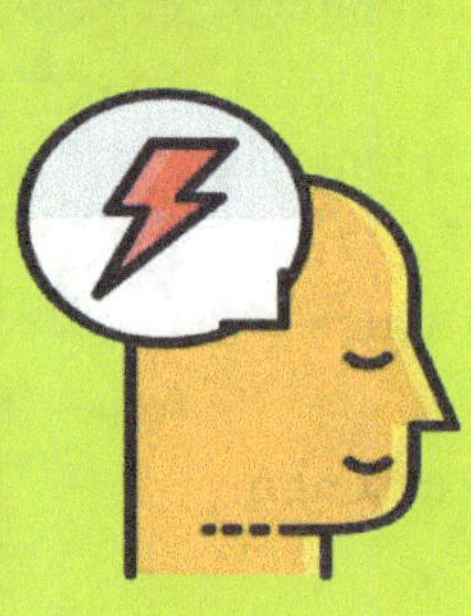

HealthyLifestyleDocs.com

WHAT'S ON THE **MIND DIET?**

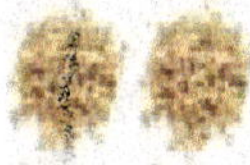 AT LEAST **THREE SERVINGS** OF WHOLE GRAINS EACH DAY

AT LEAST ONE DARK GREEN SALAD AND ONE OTHER VEGETABLE EACH DAY

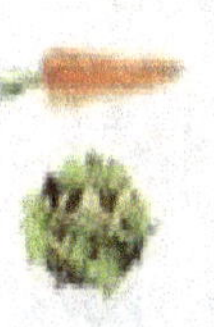

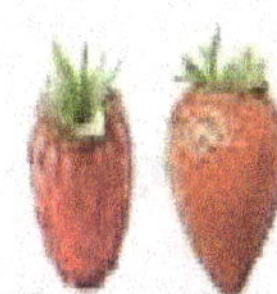 BERRIES AT LEAST TWICE A WEEK

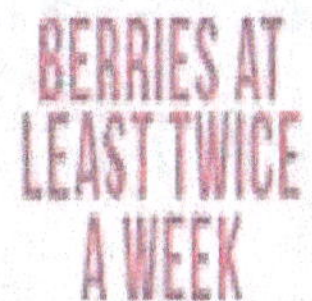 AT LEAST A ONE-OUNCE SERVING OF NUTS EACH DAY 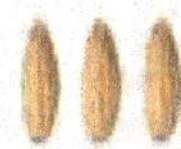

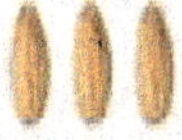

BEANS OR LEGUMES AT LEAST EVERY OTHER DAY

POULTRY AT LEAST TWICE A WEEK

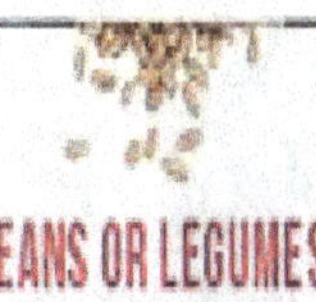

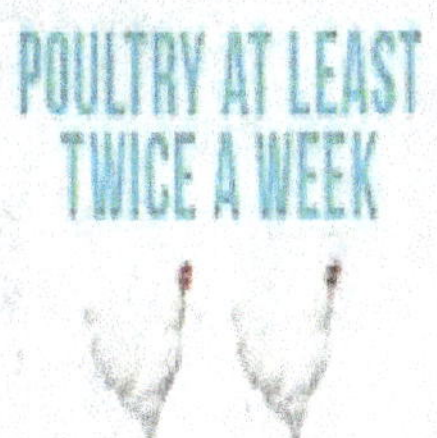 FISH AT LEAST ONCE A WEEK

If you don't drink alcohol, purple grape juice provides many of the same benefits.

A FIVE-OUNCE GLASS OF RED WINE EACH DAY 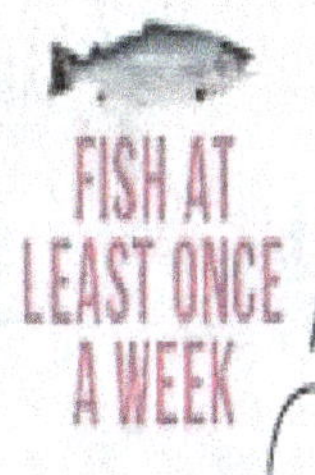

NO MORE THAN ONE TABLESPOON A DAY OF BUTTER OR MARGARINE; CHOOSE OLIVE OIL INSTEAD

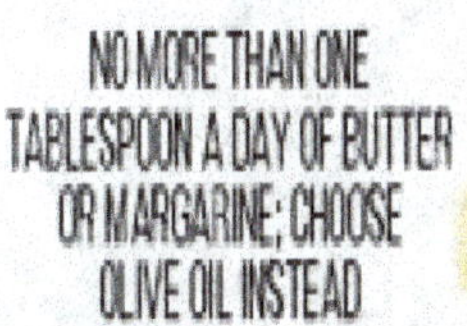

 CHEESE, FRIED FOOD AND FAST FOOD NO MORE THAN ONCE A WEEK

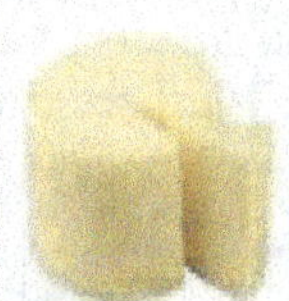

PASTRIES AND SWEETS LESS THAN FIVE TIMES A WEEK 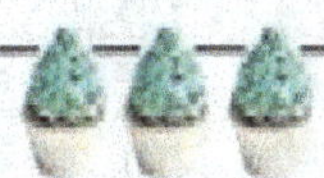

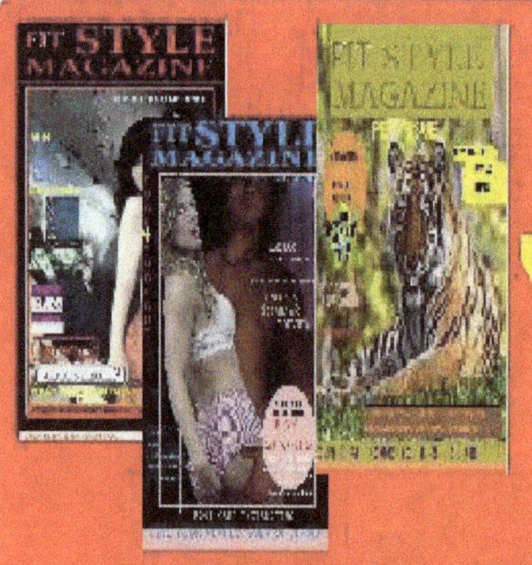

CELEB- PET- MUSIC-HEALTH

LOCAL-REGIONAL-NATIONAL-WORLDWIDE

CONTACT-937-848-0342

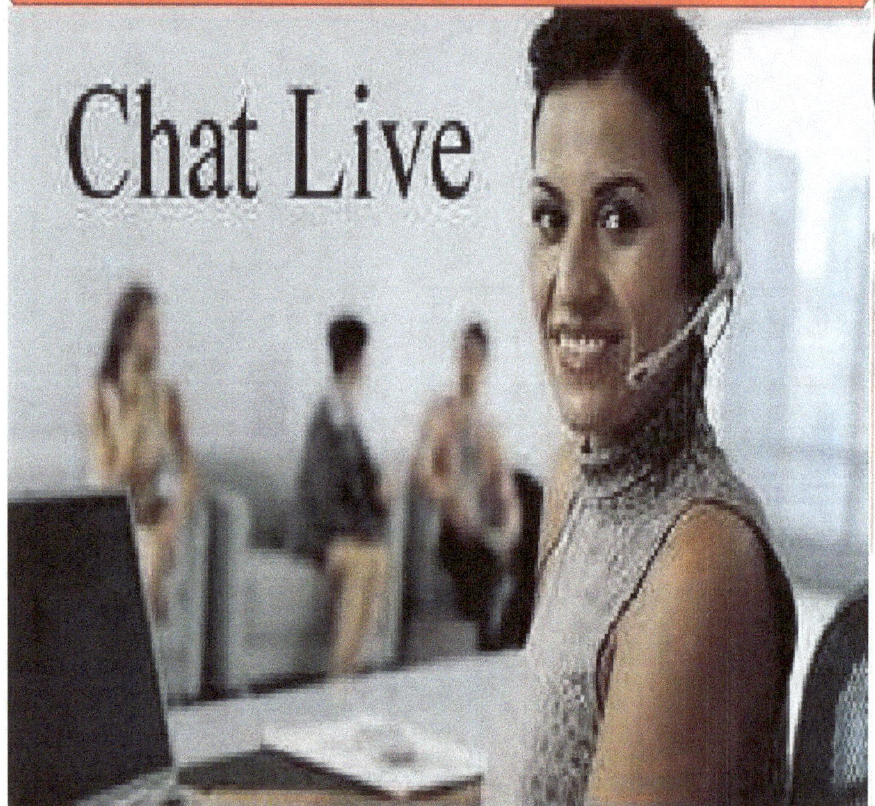

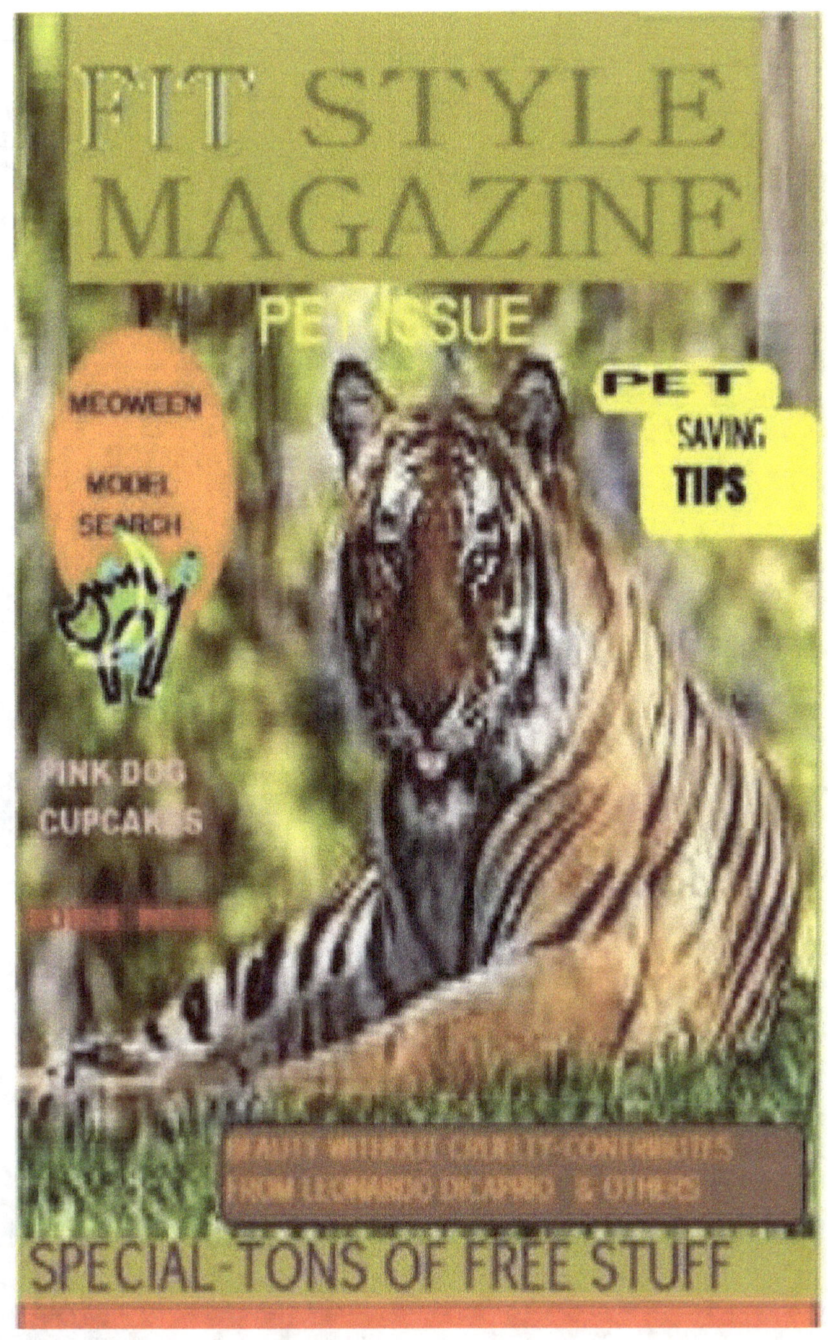

SPECIAL CONTRIBUTION FROM LEONARDO DICAPRIO
BUY TO HELP RAISE AWARENESS FREE STUFF FOR YOUR FAVORITE FURR
FRIENDS FROM SPONSORS ALL OVER.INSIDE.
SOME MAY HAVE EXPIRED UPDATES ARE REVISED WHEN CAN

Shop normally. Nothing to remember. Over 1,400 favorite stores & the iGive Button make helping easy, free, and automatic.

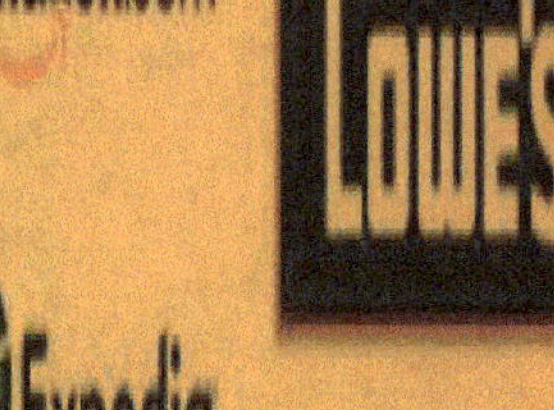

amazon.com
LOWE'S
Crate&Barrel

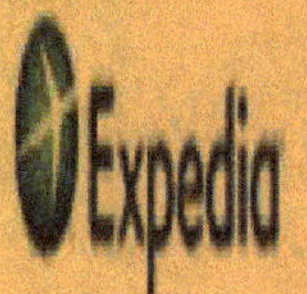

Expedia
Walgreens

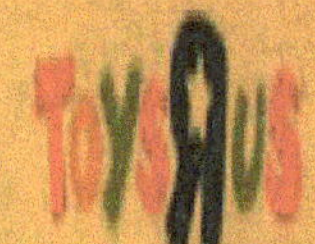

macy's
STAPLES

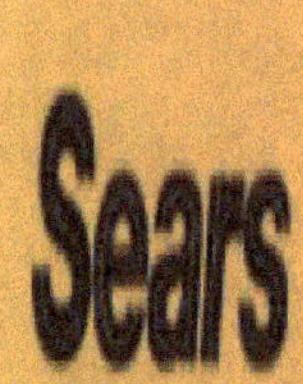

Toys "R" Us
KOHL'S

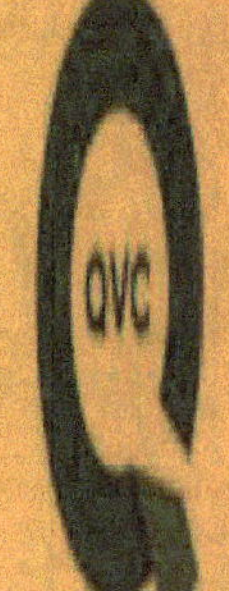

qvc
PETCO
Where the pets go.

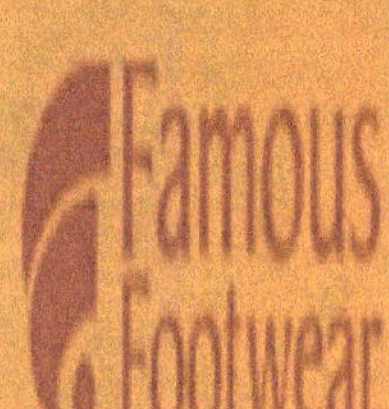

Sears
Famous Footwear

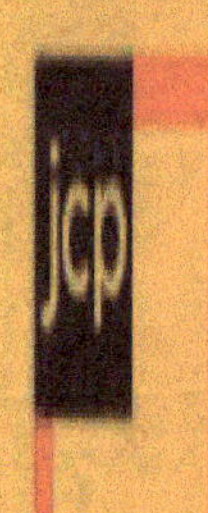

jcp

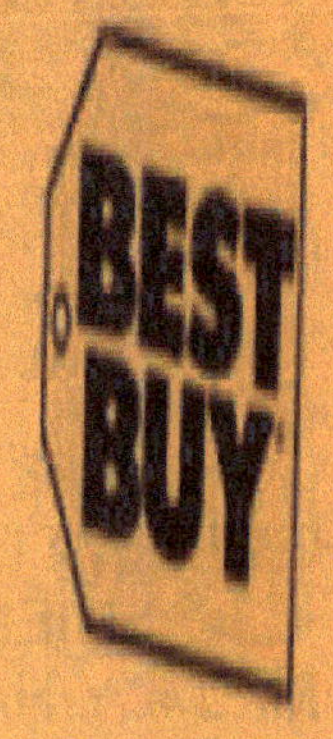

BED BATH & BEYOND
ORBITZ
BEST BUY

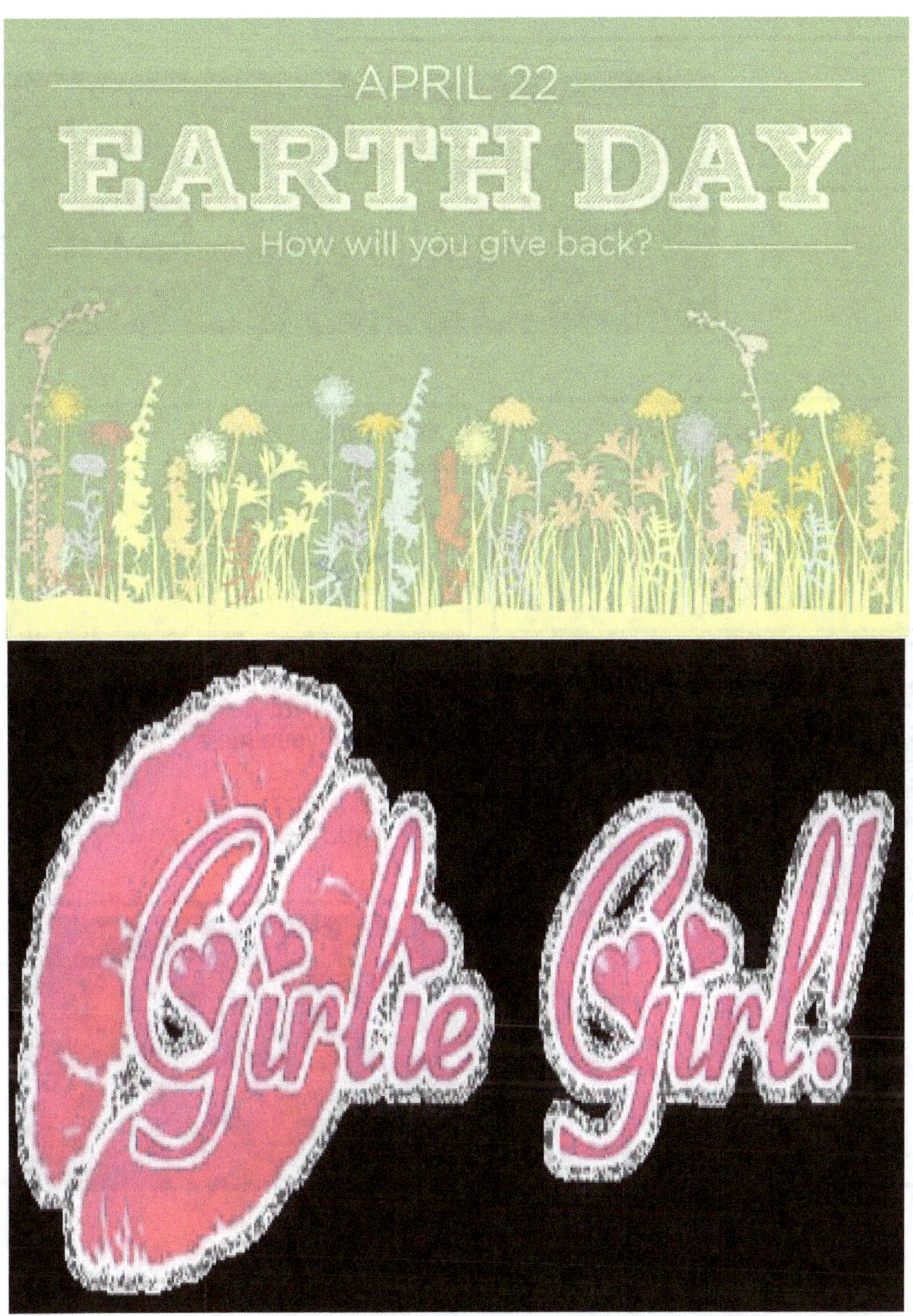

Magazine visit www.girliegirllove.blogspot.com

FITSTYLE MAGAZINE WANTS TO SPONSOR YOU!

HOW DOES THAT SOUND?

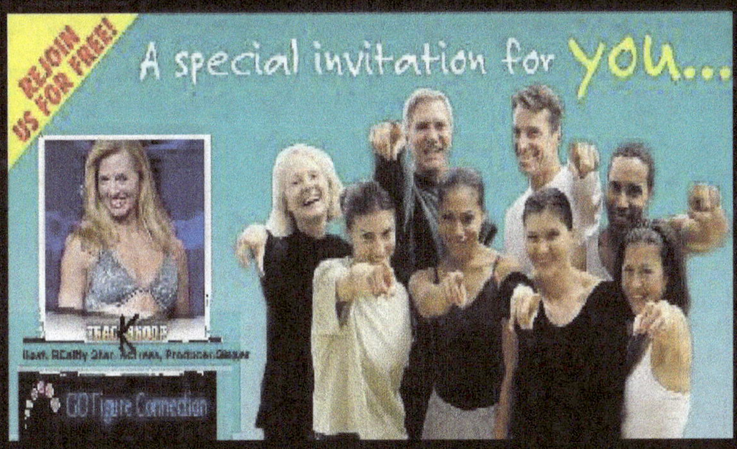

STEP 1- GO TO
WWW.FITPROLIFESTYLE.WEBS.COM
STEP 2- REGISTER
STEP 3- ANSWER SOME QUESTIONS AND
UPLOAD SOME PHOTOS
STEP 4-INVITE EVERYONE YOU KNOW TO VIEW
YOUR PROFILE AND JOIN.
STEP 5-SUBMIT ARTICLES AND CHANCE TO BE
FEATURED IN THE MAGAZINE ......MEMBERS

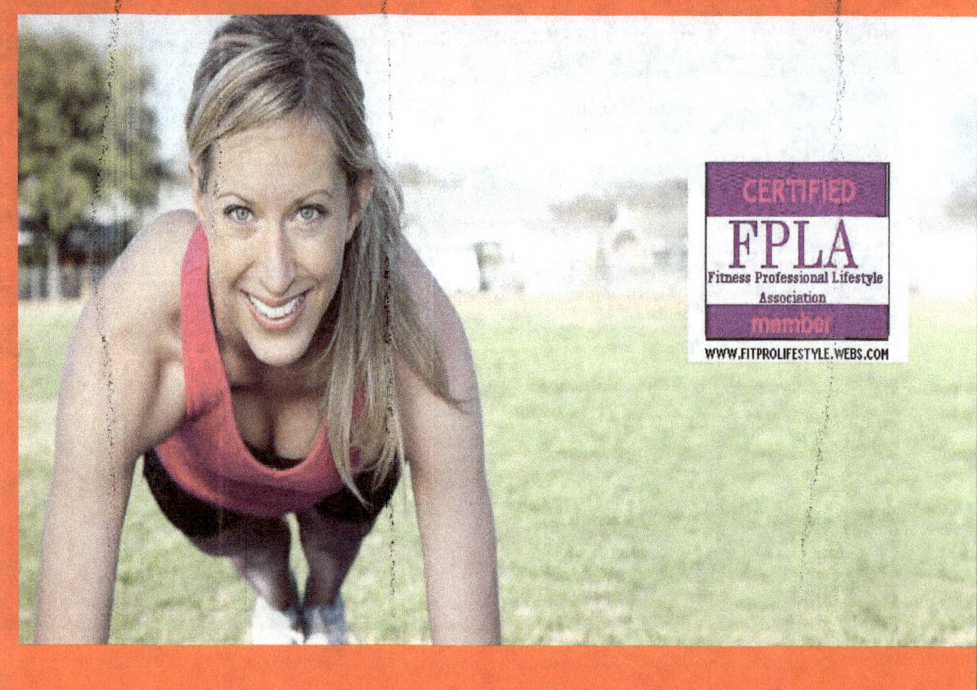

GO FIT GO PRO GET A LIFESTYLE

WITH FPLA - BENEFITS ARE GROWING

WHY SHOULDN'T YOU GET REWARDED

CERTIFIED
FPLA
Fitness Professional Lifestyle
Association
member
WWW.FITPROLIFESTYLE.WEBS.COM

Contact us for advertising rates and a media kit

WE NEED YOUR ADVERTISING DOLLARS

Target Market

Income level averaging $50,000

Target audience levels

25-45 ages

13-25 ages

Over 45

Military

Fashion

Models

Beauty

Reality and Celebs

Following of close to half a million with founder

Subscribers 10,000

Sponsorship packages start at $2500

Contact us by email.   Send your info to apply for

Membership…

Annual contracts welcomed…for bids

Email our VA's Linda or Jen on the site for an appointment

Free consultation …service fees vary

www.ingramcontent.com/pod-product-compliance
Lightning Source LLC
Chambersburg PA
CBHW081833250726
48657CB00019B/3164